The Four Treasures of Tai Chi and Qigong:

Developing Essence, Energy, Spirit, and Power Through Chi Movements

ChiFusion™ Tai Chi and Qigong

Al J. Simon

DISCLAIMER AND/OR LEGAL NOTICES:

The practices described in this work are for information purposes only, and neither the author nor the publisher shall be held liable or responsible for any harm to anyone from the direct or indirect application of the knowledge or ideas expressed in the work. This work refers to traditional health, healing, and energy systems, and there are no claims for their effectiveness. Please consult a physician and/or health professional before engaging in any physical activity or before taking any advice from this work.

First Printing, 2018

ISBN: 9781720168669

In This Book

In this book, you'll discover:

- **How to "de-mystify" your Tai Chi and Qigong with practical, tangible explanations. (page 2)**

- What are the "four treasures" of Tai Chi and Qigong? (page 7)

- **What EXACTLY is chi, and does it really exist? (page 13)**

- Why we don't define chi just as "energy" - instead here's an experiential definition of chi. (page 15)

- **How your instructors can help you experience chi ... and why it's their responsibility. (page 16)**

- The "bravery" of chi, and the importance of "unabstracting" the four treasures. (page 18)

- **The "process/activity/result" mindset used by Tai Chi, Qigong, and traditional Chinese medicine. (page 19)**

- The one scientifically measurable component of chi that proves it's not all in your head. (page 23)

- **What is "jing" (essence) and how does it affect our health? (page 25)**

- How "pre-birth jing" creates a special focus on the internal organs in Tai Chi and Qigong. (page 27)

- What are the three "post-birth jing" processes we should focus on for health and energy? (page 29)

- Four "post-birth jing" breathing practices that can be done at any time to boost your chi production. (page 32)

- The importance of "detailed regulating" for chi cultivation in Tai Chi and Qigong. (page 39)

- Where one-size-fits-all, "monkey-see, monkey-do" chi practices fail, and how they need to be "custom fitted" to your body, mind, and energy system. (page 43)

- Eight ways to regulate your body to improve your chi development. (page 45)

- The relationship between "shen" (spirit) and "yun shui" ("cloud-water") mind. (page 61)

- The relationship between shen cultivation and other disciplines like Taoism and Zen. (page 62)

- Cultivating shen mindfulness to quiet the inner programming of the "monkey mind." (page 64)

- Practicing silent Qigong as a way to cultivate shen. (page 67)

- Why most "chi limitations" aren't physical, and how one of our wheelchair bound students proved it. (page 73)

- Why you can't change your chi development without affecting your body, mind, and emotions. (page 77)

- The relationship between chi development and shen development. (page 78)

- Five "tips from the masters" on developing the right shen mindset for chi development. (page 80)

- The skeptical, "non-believer" attitude encouraged by a 103-year-old Tai Chi master (page 81)

- Why the world's most famous martial artist encouraged "breaking away from forms and formulas" in your practice (page 83)

- How a former U.S. national champion approaches questions and problems in his Tai Chi and Qigong. (page 85)

- The advice from a Zen master, and the Tai Chi version of that advice, that shows the limitations of prior learning. (page 87).

- A dramatic example of "beginner's mind" in action that I personally witnessed between to famous martial artists. (page 89)

- The single biggest "mental skill" you need for high level chi development. (page 94)

- The real meaning of "wei wu wei" (effortless action) from the Taoist path. (page 98)

- Why yin and yang are so misunderstood even among Chinese, and the original meanings of the terms. (page 134)

- **An everyday example shows how yin and yang are "relative" to our sensory organs. (page 136)**

- The three "instructional methods" in Tai Chi and Qigong, and how they use yin and yang. (page 139)

- **The "inner warrior" - using your natural reactions in a conflict situation (page 153)**

- How "natural reactions" are worked into most Tai Chi forms. (page 157)

- **Examples of each of the four intentional reactions in Tai Chi. (page 160)**

- From intention to internal power: the relationship of four elemental intentions to Tai Chi's "eight energies." (page 169)

- **The structural aspects of internal power, and why they are important. (page 181)**

- Why "combat jin" sometimes interferes with "healthy jin". (page 182)

- **Five body skills needed to express "four elements jin." (page 185).**

- The chi pyramid: how to develop a lesson plan for developing chi and jin from scratch. (page 189)

Contents

Your Invitation

Want to learn more advanced approaches and practices in Chi Development?

We invite you to join us as we explore how to break through to higher levels of health, stress relief, vitality, energy, and power in your Tai Chi and Qigong practice.

For support in taking your next steps towards higher levels in your Tai Chi and Qigong, please visit us online at:

www.QiMasters.com

Al J. Simon

"De-Mystifying" Your Tai Chi and Qigong

Confused About How Chi Development Really Works?

"You are About to Discover the Real Theory Behind Chi Development - REVEALED in Practical, Everyday Language for Experienced Students and Instructors."

Many Tai Chi instructors include "chi theory" in their teaching, but usually with vague, confusing explanations.

But starting today, I'm going to show you how to relate this to YOUR Tai Chi and Qigong, with easy-to-follow, practical examples.

Dear Friend –

Would you like to really understand the theory behind Qigong and Tai Chi - not in vague, hypothetical terms - but in practical, easy-to-understand language?

Would you like to know how this theory relates directly to your practice, your health, and your Chi Development?

You may already know that many Tai Chi and Qigong instructors include "theoretical" material in their teaching. Unfortunately though, this theory is often presented in a disconnected fashion from your actual practice.

For example, an instructor might tell you that in Tai Chi and Qigong, "*jing* creates chi." Then they will teach you the movements of their Tai Chi and Qigong style.

But do they ever point out exactly how the movements cause "*jing*" to create "chi"?

Do they point out EXACTLY where and how it happens?

And even worse, I've even heard instructors say that you just have to take these theories "on faith". You have to believe in chi, in *jing*, or in these other concepts - and believe that the theory is what's happening in Tai Chi and Qigong. "*Just trust me, it's happening*", as I once heard one teacher say at a workshop to about 40 students.

But wouldn't you rather have useful explanations - not some nice theories that you have to take on faith - but practical and tangible explanations that are directly applicable to what you are learning in Tai Chi and Qigong?

The Fast Track to Understanding Chi

Hi, I'm Al Simon. I'm a certified Tai Chi and Qigong Master, recognized by the Headfounders Grandmasters Council and the International Martial Arts Council of America.

In addition, I've been inducted into the United States Martial Arts Hall of Fame three times - as a Master and a Founder for my contributions to Tai Chi and Qigong.

I've been practicing the ancient arts of Tai Chi and Qigong over the last 30 years. I learned my first Qigong exercises back in 1975 (back when it was called "Chinese yoga"), and began learning Tai Chi in 1984.

Over the last 20 years, I've taught a comprehensive system of chi life energy development called ChiFusion™ Tai Chi and Qigong.

This system contains many practical exercises to help people improve their health, relieve stress, gain balance and flexibility, recover from illness and disease, and develop energy and vitality.

At the time of this writing, over 4,500 students around the world have benefited from our Complete Course in ChiFusion™ Tai Chi and Qigong.

We've received many emails from them thanking us for finally showing them how to feel chi for themselves - simply, directly, and easily.

Explore Practical Chi Theory

Our ChiFusion™ Tai Chi and Qigong system contains many practical exercises for Chi Development. While we do cover some theory in our courses, mostly we focus on exercises you could use to develop chi for yourself, rather than presenting a lot of theory.

However, many of our ChiFusion™ students told us they wanted to know more about the theory behind these exercises. And knowing how much we strive to "de-mystify" Tai Chi, Qigong, and Chi Development, they have asked us for more practical, direct explanations and applications of these theories.

Well, we listened to them - and we've put together this special 200+ page book designed to de-mystify the theory behind Tai Chi and Qigong.

Theory That Relates to Your Practice

This special book you now hold in your hands, entitled "The Four Treasures of Tai Chi and Qigong," discusses the theory behind Tai Chi and Qigong in clear, easy-to-understand language.

We've written this book specifically for intermediate and advanced students and instructors of all styles of Qigong and Tai Chi. This theory relates directly to the practices you are learning and teaching in your classes and courses.

To create this book, we've compiled some of our best teachings that cover the *Three Treasures of Chinese Medicine,* their relation to Tai Chi and Qigong, and their relation to the *Internal Power* of Tai Chi.

Plus, we've added new material on the topics of *Internal Power (jin) and the Eight Energies of Tai Chi* that has not appeared in our courses or books before. This is material that we've taught in classes and workshops since the mid-1990's, but has never appeared in print before!

Not For Beginners

I should point out that this book is not for beginners.

In this book, I assume that you have at least some experience with Tai Chi or Qigong. The more experience you have, the better.

So if you have <u>no</u> experience, or if you are a beginner who has taken only a few classes, this book may not be right for you.

Instead, for new students, I'd recommend starting with my *Qigong Self-Massage and Chi Washing* book. It's a beginner-friendly introduction to Chi Development that will help you get started the right way. You'll find it at <u>www.ChiWashing.com</u>.

But if you are an intermediate or advanced student of Qigong and Tai Chi who wants to challenge themselves by going deeper into Chi Development, you are in the right place.

So let's get started ...

I hope you find this book valuable, and I wish you all the best in your exploration of Chi Development.

Best wishes,
Al Simon

Certified Tai Chi and Qigong Master, Three-time Inductee into the U.S. Martial Arts Hall of Fame

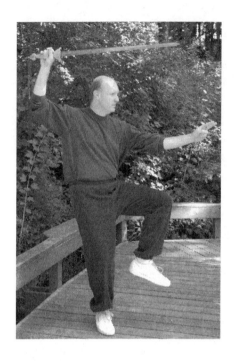

What are the Four Treasures?

This all started one day when one of our ChiFusion™ students sent me this message:

Dear Al,

I am new to ChiFusion™ Tai Chi and Qigong and may seem to be asking an advanced question. But they seem to lead to necessary experiences in the realm of internal arts.

I am looking forward to making progress in the courses and like what I see so far and what I have gotten so far has been great.

I have been practicing various forms of Tai Chi and Chi Kung [Qigong] for a while and do feel the chi in my practice. I love learning new material that communicates from the marrow of the practice, not just forms.

*I am interested to hear what you have to say about the relation of the development of chi to **the development of jin or internal power as well as jing, chi, and shen to emptiness transformations**. Also, if you have any insight into the relation of jin, internal power, to jing, one of the three treasures.*

Thanks in advance.

Bill

While I answered Bill's question briefly in a return message, what grew out of his question was a series of articles in our newsletter. This series discussed the Three Treasures of Chinese Medicine, their relation to Tai Chi and Qigong, and their relation to Tai Chi's approach to Internal Power.

Normally in our courses and books, we focus first and foremost on the practical side of Chi Development.

While we do cover some theory in our courses, we generally avoid theoretical discussions. Instead, we stack our courses with practical "exercises" and "experiments" you can use to develop Chi. We do cover some theory. But we do so only when it is absolutely necessary for you to understand the purposes and the benefits of the exercises and movements you are learning.

But mostly, we focus on exercises you could try to feel "Chi" for yourself, rather than having to "understand" or "believe in" theories.

By focusing on the practical, we've found that you can get health, stress relief, and Chi Development benefits much more quickly than if we padded our books (and your brain!) with theory.

A vast majority of our students prefer it this way. At the time of this writing, over 4,500 students around the world have benefited from our course in Chi Development.

In addition, a select group of students and instructors have gone on to join us in our *Qi Masters* program, where we explore the details of Chi Development in all its intricate details.

As a result, we've received many emails from our students and instructors thanking us for this "direct" approach.

However, a number of our students like Bill, who've learned from other teachers, have heard these theories before and wanted to know more about them.

So here was my answer to Bill, which I published on our forum and in our newsletters.

It explains briefly the Four Treasures in a straight-forward fashion. Take this answer as an overview of the topics, before we delve into more details in the rest of this book.

Dear Bill -

Thank you for your question.

First, for those unfamiliar with the terms, here are some brief explanations:

Jing, **chi, and** *shen* are considered the Three Treasures of Traditional Chinese Medicine.

"*Jing*" **is the name given to the "raw material"** from which we create life-energy called "chi." This raw material consists of genetically acquired material (pre-birth *jing*), plus the raw material acquired from food, drink, breathing, and chi cultivation practices (post-birth *jing*).

This raw material is converted to life-energy (chi). With further practice and cultivation, chi may be converted (though "refined" is a better word) to "*shen*".

"*Shen*" **is often roughly translated as "spirit",** but probably "higher awareness" or "personal realization" may be better translations.

9

Those in a nutshell are the Three Treasures of Chinese Medicine, so let's move on to the concept of *"jin."*

Jin **is often translated as "internal power" or "intrinsic energy".** In its widest possible definition, it refers to the outward expression of our cultivation of "chi" and "*shen*" to the world around us.

In martial arts and Tai Chi, *jin* often narrowly refers to the expression of "chi" to generate power in movement. In more spiritually-oriented disciplines, *jin* may refer to how we use our "higher awareness" to reach even higher levels in our path to the highest level of "personal enlightenment" or "emptiness".

Taken together, you can look at the Three Treasures of Chinese Medicine (*jing*, chi, and *shen*) along with *jin* as **the Four Treasures of Tai Chi and Qigong.**

Many consider these Four Treasures as some of the "basic theory" upon which Tai Chi and Qigong are built.

However, if you look through our courses and books, you'll find us mentioning "chi", but you won't find us mentioning *jing, shen,* or *jin.*

Why?

The most practical reason we don't use these terms is the same reason we avoid most Chinese terms in our course: **clarity**.

In developing our course, we wanted to **de-mystify the process** of understanding Tai Chi and Qigong as much as possible for English speakers. We still use a handful of Chinese words (*dantien, kua,* and *laogong* leap to mind) where we had difficulty finding English equivalents.

A second reason is that we want you to **focus more on the transformations** among *jing*, chi, *shen*, and *jin*, rather than on these things as separate entities.

For example, we don't want you to think of "*jing*" and "chi" as two separate things, but to think of "*jing*-to-chi" as a process.

Now combine this "process-oriented" view along with our attempt to render information in English. Given those two reasons, in our course **you can start to see examples where we are talking about transformations without using those words.**

For example, you'll find many places where we talk about "activating", "stimulating", or "revving up". Those are some of the terms we use to discuss the "*jing*-to-chi" process. You can find similar equivalents for the "chi-to-*shen*" process, the "chi-and-*shen*-to-*jin*" process, and the "*jin*-to-emptiness" process.

A third reason that we rarely mention these terms - and probably the most important - is due to our "Experience" method of instruction. We are much more interested in **having you be able to do these transformations** rather than having you just think about them. We want to teach you "intentions" rather than "theory."

Yes, we do have some theory in the course, but only enough to help you understand the intention of the exercise. Through our course, we want you to have

Al J. Simon

certain experiences like the transformations discussed above.

But we want you to **have these experiences in a "personal" manner, unclouded by "external" theories** of what you are supposed to experience or what is supposed to happen.

As a Zen master once said, "In the beginner's mind, there are many possibilities, but in the expert's there are few." We want you to approach these transformations with as much of a beginner's mind as possible.

Your experience and intention should always be more important than any principle or theory. Base your Tai Chi and Qigong actions on your intentions, not on principles.

If you do so, you'll reach your practice goals much more easily, and get many more benefits, whether you practice Tai Chi and Qigong for health, for chi development, or for the personal enlightenment.

Best wishes,
Al

That was my answer to Bill's question. While brief, it hits some of the highlights of theory behind *jing*, chi, *shen*, and *jin*, as well as our approach to these concepts.

So now let's fill in some of the details behind these theories, as we go through the rest of this book.

12

Energy: Does Chi Exist?

From our Four Treasures of *energy, essence, spirit, and power,* let's explore energy, which we call *chi* (sometimes spelled *qi* – pronounced "chee").

What exactly is chi?

Depending on what Tai Chi book you read, Qigong video you watch, or class you attend, you'll hear about this "mysterious energy" or "life force" that runs through our bodies called chi.

These authors/instructors usually define chi as "energy" in some fashion:

- "circulating life energy"

- "the natural energy that runs our bodies and minds"

- "the energy of the Universe, which permeates everything"

- "energy that runs along a complex series of pathways in our bodies"

- "a kind of life force or spiritual energy"

- "the very basic vital energy"

After these definitions usually comes discussions of one or more of these topics:

- Chinese medicine, history, and philosophy

- acupuncture charts and diagrams

- descriptions of fantastic martial arts feats attributed to chi

- explanations of related topics such as *feng shu*

- definitions of "energy" from other cultures

- alternative medical practices

- relating of chi to Western scientific concepts, such as quantum theory or mainstream medicine.

You might even see dramatic video of Qigong masters using chi to heal others.

You may hear how Tai Chi and Qigong are based on "theories" of chi.

If you are a Tai Chi or Qigong student, your teacher may tell you what the chi in your body is supposedly doing while you practice. Or they may tell you to "relax and use your chi" while doing Tai Chi.

But many teachers will tell you that to really experience chi, you have to "believe" in it. You have to take this theory of chi on faith. You have to believe that chi exists, and take it on faith that your Tai Chi/Qigong practice will help you develop it.

But I would like to propose a different path – one we've used successfully in our courses and programs. On this path, we follow none of those other paths to understanding chi.

Yes, we sometimes define chi as "energy", and yes, we do discuss information about "energy pathways" in our courses.

But when we get down to it, we like to define chi not in terms of "things", but in terms of "actions".

Our Definition of Chi

We like to define chi this way:

Chi is the result of performing certain "activities" and/or observing certain "processes." You can see, feel, hear, and experience chi by performing those activities and observing those processes.

This definition is extremely important, and the key to the benefits and successes our students have experienced in Tai Chi and Qigong.

We've found that defining chi as others do (as "energy"), while technically accurate, is too vague, too theoretical for our purposes. Instead, we prefer a more practical, *experiential* definition.

We define chi as "process/activity/result" to create a certain mind-set in our students. Our definition changes their perspective on chi from some vague, mystical energy (that may or may not exist, or that they may or may not experience) to something they will definitely experience by doing and observing.

Too often, instructors that define "chi as energy" place the burden of responsibility on the student. The student has to take it on faith that if they just keep practicing, they'll eventually experience chi. Unfortunately, many do keep practicing - sometimes for years - but never do experience chi.

Many instructors though fail to see how defining "chi as energy" - and the mindset it produces - can sometimes be the root of the problem.

We've found through research and student feedback that thinking of chi or any of the Four Treasures as "things" can literally block your success in experiencing them from Tai Chi and Qigong.

However, the "chi as activity" approach places the burden of responsibility for experiencing chi not on the student, **but on the instructor.**

It's up to the instructor to make sure the student learns the appropriate activities and processes. If the instructor teaches you the right things to do and observe, you will experience chi - not as some vague, mystical energy, but something you can directly feel.

If you are not experiencing chi within say the first month or two of practice, then it may simply be that the instructor is not teaching you the right things!

In the next chapter on *"jing"* or "essence", we discuss quite a bit about the actual processes that result in experiencing chi.

But before we do that, let's see how our definition of chi cuts directly through the question, "Does chi exist"?

Does Chi Exist?

As a Tai Chi and Qigong instructor, I can't count the number of times I've been asked by students in person and by email, *"Do you really believe in Chi? Is this Chi stuff real? Does Chi really exist?"*

I've also received emails from people saying, *"I don't believe in Chi. It's all in your head, or just some placebo. You'll have to prove to me that it exists."*

Of course, the assumption underlying these questions is that if chi isn't real, then we can dismiss it, and possibly dismiss its value in Tai Chi and Qigong.

Given that assumption, most of these people who ask these questions are surprised to hear what I say next.

Because I often tell them, *"Chi does NOT exist."*

"Wait a second," you may be thinking. *"You just gave us a definition of chi, and told us we can actually feel it, but now you are saying chi doesn't exist! Why the contradiction?"*

The contradiction exists when we look at "chi" (and all of the Four Treasures) not as "things," but as "abstractions".

Do you know what abstractions are?

Actually, you are quite familiar with abstractions, because all of us use them constantly in our daily lives. So before we discuss the chi as an abstraction, let's look at an example of an abstraction from daily life. It will be easier to understand *jing*, chi, *shen*, and *jin* as abstractions, if we look at something a little more familiar.

So for our real life example, let's take the concept of "bravery."

Do you know what bravery is?

A dictionary might define bravery as "a quality of spirit that enables you to face danger or pain without showing fear." Most of us would recognize bravery from this definition.

But as you know, bravery in and of itself has no shape, size, or color. It has no taste, smell, or sound. There is no "one thing" that you can point to or put your hand on and say, "this is bravery."

Bravery is not an independent object that you can detect through your five senses. Instead, bravery comes through observing certain things through your five senses, then pulling together these observations and making a summary or conclusion about them.

For example, let's say you know of someone dying of an incurable disease. Yet day after day, you see her smile and speak optimistically about the future. Or she continues to take care of her family as best as she can. Or she goes out of her way to volunteer to help others in need.

If you observed her doing these things, you might say she is showing "bravery" in the face of her illness.

Of course, what you really "see" and "hear" and "experience" are her actions. You see what she is doing, hear what she is saying, and feel how she is approaching her illness. From your observations of her actions, you "conclude" (or "interpolate" or "abstract") her bravery.

In other words, her bravery doesn't "exist" as something you can observe directly or independently of her actions. The actions are what "exists" and what you can observe. The bravery is the conclusion you draw from your observations.

The Treasures as Abstractions

In the same manner, I'd like you now to start thinking of chi and all of the Four Treasures in the same way you think of bravery.

Jing, chi, and *shen* are not things you can detect directly through your five senses. There's no "thing" you can see, taste, smell, hear, or touch that is "*jing*" or "*chi*" or "*shen*."

Instead though, you can participate in certain "activities" and observe certain "processes". And from your participation, you can draw an understanding of "chi" from what you are doing.

From a strictly disciplined "process" viewpoint, chi doesn't exist as something you can observe directly. Instead, chi can be seen, felt, and heard as an abstraction you "draw" from your experiences in Tai Chi and Qigong.

19

So how do you "draw chi"?

You perform certain "activities" and to observe certain "processes." From those activities and observations, you will experience "chi" through your observations.

Practical Applications of Abstractions

This "abstraction" approach may seem overly analytical to you. You may wonder, what difference does it make in how I think of "bravery" or "chi" or any other kind of abstraction?

Well, understanding abstractions has practical implications in any field like Tai Chi and Qigong that relates to emotional, mental, and spiritual development. And these three developments - emotional, mental, and spiritual - are the basis of *shen* transformations in Chi Development, which we will be discussing in a later chapter.

But to see an example of the practical implications of all this in a field outside of Tai Chi, look no further than psychology.

Some psychologists take special care to watch, listen, and feel when their clients use abstractions. Some therapies focus on identifying "nominalization" - an abstraction in which the client speaks about "activities" and "processes" as "things."

When clients speak in abstractions, they tend to think of their problems not as something they are "doing" but as something they "have."

Consequently, it makes it appear as if they need some sort of "treatment" to take the thing away.

Instead, the therapist tries to help the patient "un-abstract" the problem - to focus on the activity or process that is creating the problem. This gives the client the power to change their actions and create their own solutions.

To look at a classic example, a client may say to a therapist, *"I have a lot of fear; I want you to help me get rid of my fear."*

Fear, like bravery, can be regarded as an abstraction.

To help the patient "un-abstract" fear, the therapist might try to change the discussion to more process-oriented language: *"What are you afraid of? What happens while you are afraid? What are you doing when you become afraid?"*

By focusing on the persons, places, and things involved when the patient feels fear, it becomes much easier to find solutions to the actions and situations that create fear.

"Un-abstracting" Chi

Similarly, someone who asks me to prove "chi exists", or says that they are "skeptical" about chi, or wants to know how to "get chi", would benefit from this type of approach.

They need to "un-abstract" chi – that is, to stop treating it as a thing, and to change to a more process-oriented view.

That's why in Tai Chi and Qigong, we focus on processes and activities. Instead of looking at chi as a "thing," we see it as the natural result of certain well-tested activities and processes.

We work to change the student's goal from "How do I believe in chi?" or from "How do I acquire chi?" to the more process-oriented goal of "How do I make *'chi-ing'* happen?"

Far from the passive approach of many Tai Chi programs ("just keep practicing and it will happen"), through a more active approach to Tai Chi and Qigong, you gain the power to create "chi" - to really feel it - for yourself.

Now that you understand abstraction, you can easily see how Tai Chi and Qigong can help you develop "chi" - even if it doesn't exist!

For Something That Doesn't Exist, There's a Lot of It

Of course, none of this is meant to imply chi is just "all in your head." Instead, the idea here is that if you do certain things, you'll get "chi" as a result.

Moreover, there are at least some components of the "chi process" that are scientifically measurable.

For example, one of the first "chi" activities I teach students is to detect chi as it emits from the palm of their hand. This exercise allows them to actually feel chi between their hands.

If you aren't familiar with this exercise, you'll find it is in my beginners book on Chi Development, entitled *Qigong Self-Massage and Chi Washing* (available at www.ChiWashing.com.)

Far from being something mystical or imaginary, the chi emissions that beginning student feel between the palms is scientifically measurable.

Scientific research over the last few years has arrived at an explanation for chi emission in terms of infrasonic waves. Infrasonic waves are sound waves vibrating below 20 Hertz (Hz) - too slow to be audible to the human ear.

Every living person emits these waves from the palms of their hands. These waves have been measured in a number of scientific experiments and have become a well-established scientific fact. With Qigong training, we can learn to increase these waves, and also direct them through any part of our body.

In one research study, twenty-nine Americans with no prior Qigong training had the intensity of the infrasonic waves from their palms measured both before and after a week of Qigong practice. After the training, the average intensity of the waves emitted was 500% greater than before the training. And as part of the same study, one Qigong master was able to generate waves 1000 times greater than the average person emits.[1]

---

[1] [1]Lee, Richard H. "Emitted Chi Training Increases Low Frequency Sound Emission." China Healthways Institute. 5 June 1998. http://www.chi.us/researchemitedchi.htm (7 July 2018).

Adding to these studies, Western medicine is exploring the value of distance healing methods that include therapeutic touch - using healing energy in the hands - when working with patients.[2]

In the long run, therapeutic touch and chi emission may actually involve more than just infrasonic waves. But the fact that at least one component of chi can be measured suggests that chi emission, like chi itself, is more than just part of our imagination.

But certainly, the most effective way to approach chi is to realize that it is the result of certain processes and activities.

So what are these processes and activities you can use to observe chi?

---

[2] Astin, John A, Elaine Harkness, and Edzard Ernst. "The Efficacy of 'Distant Healing': A Systematic Review of Randomized Trials." Annals of Internal Medicine. Vol. 132 No. 11. 6 June 2000. https://annals.org/aim/article-abstract/713514/efficacy-distant-healing-systematic-review-randomized-trials (7 July 2018).

Essence: The Power of *Jing*

So far, we've discussed how the benefits of Tai Chi and Qigong are built on the "Three Treasures" of Traditional Chinese Medicine - namely *jing*, chi, and *shen*.

And in the last chapter, we pointed out that chi (and this applies as well to *jing* and *shen*) is not a "thing" you "have." Instead, *jing*, chi, and *shen* are the results of certain processes you can observe and certain activities in which you can participate.

So what are these processes and activities you can use to observe chi?

Well, the most important processes start with an exploration of the first Treasure, *jing* or Essence. Many Qigong and Tai Chi masters consider *jing* as the most important to properly cultivate for your overall physical, emotional, and spiritual health.

As we've mentioned before, *jing* is the name given to the "raw material" from which we create life-energy called "chi."

This raw material consists of genetically acquired material known as *pre-birth jing,* plus the raw material acquired from food, drink, breathing, and chi cultivation practices, known as *post-birth jing.*

The Processes of Pre-Birth *Jing*

Though I've used the term "material" in describing *jing*, remember to think not in terms of "things" but in terms of "processes".

For example, "pre-birth *jing*" is not a separate entity or "thing" you have in your body. A doctor can't open you up surgically and point to your pre-birth *jing*.

Instead, think of pre-birth *jing* as an abstract term that refers to the results of the activity of all of the internal processes that happen in your body.

The "pre-birth *jing*" processes range from the microscopic (your DNA, chemical bonding and hormonal secretions in your body fluids, the absorption of nutrients in your digestive system) to the macroscopic (internal structure and function of your organs, your skeletal structure, and your nervous system).

The basic "rhythm" and "functioning" of these pre-birth *jing* processes inside your body were set at birth, based on the genetics of your parents.

Pre-Birth *Jing* in Tai Chi and Qigong

Tai Chi and Qigong students place special emphasis on the organ functioning aspects of the pre-birth *jing* processes. Much of the beginning work in high-level Tai Chi and Qigong focuses on your internal organs through both static and moving Qigong.

As an example, let's take a simple exercise like *Raise Heels* from Eight Brocades Qigong. This is often the first exercise we teach to new Tai Chi and Qigong students.

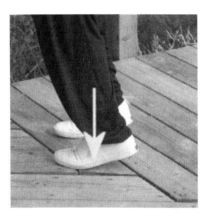

This exercise is done by simply raising the heels off the ground just enough to put pressure on the *Bubbling Well* acupuncture point in the foot.

The *Bubbling Well* is located in the hollow depression just behind the ball of the foot between the metatarsals of the second and third toes. The name of this point comes from the fact that it is our primary energetic connection with the earth, and that energy "bubbles up" from the wellspring of the earth into this point.

This point is the also known as *KI-1*, since it is the first point on the Kidney energy meridian.

In other words, this point primarily focuses on the kidneys in the body.

Generally, when you are first starting out in Tai Chi and Qigong that emphasizes the Four Treasures, you'll find that nearly every exercise targets specific internal organs and/or processes like this one does.

You'll find yourself working to improve the *jing* provided by all of your primary internal organs: kidneys, spleen, liver, stomach, gall bladder, bladder, intestines, lungs, and heart. You'll also find improvements in your internal processes of the circulatory, respiratory, digestive, elimination, immune, lymphatic, reproductive, and nervous systems.

In the beginning work of high-level Tai Chi and Qigong, we place special emphasis on directly affecting the kidneys.

According to traditional Chinese medicine, the kidneys are the most important organs in our body. This statement may seem odd to Westerners, who usually think of the heart or lungs as the most important organs. But in Chinese medicine, Qigong, Tai Chi, and acupuncture, the kidneys **directly influence the conversion of *jing* to internal chi energy.**

Keep in mind that in Western medicine, when we refer to the kidneys, we are talking about specific organs, that is, specific "things". But in Chinese medicine - with its greater emphasis on "processes" rather than "things" - when we say "kidneys," we are not referring just to the kidney organs. We're referring to the entire uro-genital process involved in reproduction as well as waste elimination.

The Chinese consider the uro-genital process to be the foundation of life and internal energy. And it literally is, given its involvement in reproduction. As a matter of fact, "*jing*" is sometimes translated as "sperm", though the association of "*jing*" with sexual reproduction is more symbolic than actual.

Because of the importance of the kidneys, especially in the beginning work of high-level Tai Chi and Qigong, many of the beginning lessons specifically focus on the kidneys. So it's no wonder that even a simple exercise like *Raise Heels* focuses on an acupuncture point associated with the *pre-birth jing* in the kidneys.

Three Processes of Post-Birth *Jing*

As we mentioned, the basic "rhythm" and "functioning" of the internal processes inside your body were set at birth, based on the genetics of your parents.

For most of us, the inherited internal processes of pre-birth *jing* can at times place certain limits on our overall health.

We've all heard of or seen children that were born "health poor", for whom life is a struggle right from the start. And we also have heard of the "health rich" who live long lives into their 90's and beyond <u>without</u> ever exercising or dieting, and often engaging in known health-risky behavior such as smoking.

It may seem unfair, but we are all born with a certain amount of health. That is our "pre-birth *jing*". Health-poor individuals struggle with health from the start. Health-rich individuals never have to worry about their health.

Most of us though fall between these two extremes when it comes to pre-birth *jing*. Most of us are born with a certain amount of health that for the average person, lasts anywhere from 20 to 50 years. Once that genetically-inherited health runs out, usually toward middle age, we start to experience problems that seem to "come out of nowhere".

Traditional Chinese Medicine (abbreviated TCM) recognizes that we inherit a limited amount of health that sustains us in our early years, then runs out as we age.

However, TCM points out that **we can compensate for this genetic and age-related limitation by our choices of "post-birth *jing*" processes.** Post-birth *jing* processes can be used to overcome these limitations and increase our health significantly.

Post-birth *jing* includes three internal processes over which we have outside control: **digestion, respiration, and chi cultivation.**

Post-Birth *Jing* #1: Digestion

There is no doubt that the first "post-birth *jing*" process - what we eat and drink - affects our health. These days, who hasn't heard about the health implications – both good and bad – of what we eat.

But despite all the advances of modern dietary science, there seems to be little agreement among so-called "diet experts" about what constitutes a healthy diet.

The reason there is so little agreement?

Most diet experts fail to account for "pre-birth *jing*" differences - those genetic dispositions that make the same diet healthy for one person, but damaging to another.

For example, at times high-protein diets have been the rage here in the United States. When that happened, many people jumped on the high-protein bandwagon and were eating lots of protein.

While a number of people are thriving on this type of diet, obesity in our country continues to rise. Why? Because only a certain percentage of people have the right genetics for a high-protein diet. For the rest of us, a high-protein diet will throw off our metabolic processes, causing all sorts of health problems.

And that's true of any diet. A vegan diet will work great for one person, but actually be damaging to the physical health of another person. It's not the diet though. It's the pre-birth *jing* of the dieter that makes the diet right or wrong for them.

A low-fat diet, as another example, will improve the health of a certain percentage of people, while causing weight gain, sickness, and a drain on pre-birth *jing* for others. Yes, it may be hard to believe, but a low-fat diet will cause you to gain weight if it is incompatible with your pre-birth *jing*.

Diet is a complex topic - much more complex than we can cover in this book. But as a general recommendation, there are a number of approaches to eating that specialize in how genetic factors determine proper diet.

Some look at a limited number of genetic factors, like the "blood type" diets or the "hair analysis" diets that were the rage a few years ago. But the more genetic factors you look at, the more likely you are to find the right diet for you. I recommend starting with something like a *metabolic typing* or a diet approach that looks at a wide variety of genetic factors.

But whatever diet approach you consider, make sure it includes methods and approaches for *customizing* the diet to make it fit your unique mind, body, and energy system.

Post-Birth *Jing* #2: Respiration

The second post-birth *jing* process - how we breathe - can have dramatic effects on our health. Proper breathing improves health, relieves stress, and aids in Chi development.

Have you ever watched a baby breathe? A baby's whole torso expands with each breath. The baby is oxygenating her body to help maintain good health and strong growth during these critical early years.

Unfortunately, by the time that baby is an adult, she most likely will be taking shallow breaths that will ruin her health and well-being!

Did you know that the first part of our body affected by lack of oxygen is the brain? It consumes 20% of the available oxygen in each breath. So if our breathing is shallow, we are literally breathing ourselves "stupid."

As a matter of fact, some have suggested that old-age forgetfulness not related to Alzheimer's Disease may actually be due to decades of oxygen starvation to the brain!

So what can you do? Begin by unlearning those "lazy breathing" habits, and get back to the deep way you breathed as a baby!

But proper breathing involves much more than just taking "deep breaths." In Qigong and Tai Chi, we have many different breathing techniques beyond the simple "deep breathing" level. Because of this, I consider proper breathing a foundation upon which you can build your own personal Chi Development.

Briefly, here are some breathing techniques you can use. You can use these during your Qigong and Tai Chi practice, but they also make great stand-alone practices as well.

Post-Birth Breathing Method 1: Natural Breathing

Natural breathing is the first practice you should start with, before attempting any of the other type of Tai Chi or Qigong breathing.

It is also the simplest practice to learn. As the name implies, natural breathing is merely breathing as you normally breathe. The practice is merely to become consciously aware of your current breathing pattern.

Take a short period of time, two minutes or three minutes to start, and simply become aware of your breathing. Do not try to change your breathing pattern. Simply spend a few quiet minutes trying to become aware of how you currently breathe.

While simple to learn, practicing natural breathing is more difficult than it sounds.

Post-Birth Breathing Method 2: Normal Abdominal Breathing

Normal abdominal breathing is breathing deeply into the lower lungs and diaphragm. When we ask new students to take a deep breath, many of them expand their chest and even raise their shoulders as they inhale. That's not what we mean by a deep breath. That's a full shallow breath. In contrast, during a deep breath, the lower belly expands as you inhale. The chest and shoulders move very little or not at all.

Note that the stomach does not expand from moving the stomach muscles. Instead you completely relax the stomach muscles.

As you inhale, direct the breath into the lower lungs. The stomach will expand all on its own if you keep it relaxed.

As you exhale, you continue to keep the stomach relaxed and allow the stomach to return to its normal relaxed position.

For abdominal breathing, start with very short practice times – no more than one to two minutes to begin with. Inhale only to 70% of your capacity.

Also, only practice for about 70% of the maximum time you can practice. So for example, if you think you can do three minutes of abdominal breathing, only practice for about two minutes (about 70% of the maximum time).

If you feel light-headed or dizzy during this practice, you've gone over your 70% (and possibly your 100%) in either amount of practice time or amount of inhale. If so, immediately discontinue practice.

Post-Birth Breathing Method 3: Reverse Abdominal Breathing

In the normal abdominal breathing practice above, you kept your stomach relaxed. In reverse abdominal breathing, you actually do use your stomach muscles and move your abdomen. But you move your abdomen in the opposite direction to normal abdominal breathing.

In reverse ab breathing, as you inhale, you pull your abdomen in towards you. As you exhale, you push it out away from you.

I'm using the terms "pull" and "push" but this should be done in as relaxed a manner as possible. We're not looking for big contractions and expansions. Use only a small movement, with minimal effort.

This exercise can be a bit more taxing on the bodymind, so I suggest using the 40% level for the stomach movement instead of 70%.

In other words, only contract and expand your stomach to 40% of the most you can move your stomach muscles. I still keep to 40% today, even though I'm healthy and experienced with this practice.

If you are new, you may want to do only 10% or 20% to start, and work up to 40%. Start with only one minute of practice. If you feel light-headed, or if you find your pulse racing, or sense any other "pressures" or "forcing" inside your body, discontinue practice.

Post-Birth Breathing Method 4: Thin Breathing

Thin breathing is usually done with a relaxed stomach like normal abdominal breathing. But the air is taken in very slowly, not with a big inhale, but with a slow, relaxed inhale. The breath is also released slowly with a small exhale.

In thin breathing, the key ideas are **deep, slow, thin, and quiet.**

Deep refers to allowing the breath to be drawn down into the lower lungs, just as with normal ab breathing.

Slow refers to slowing down the breathing process, taking much longer than usual to inhale and exhale.

For example, if you normally inhale for five seconds and exhale for five seconds, you'll want to expand that time. You might start by doing a seven or ten second inhale, followed by a seven to ten second exhale. Over time, you'll want to work at slowing down the breath even more.

Thin refers to breathing in a small, continuous unbroken stream, so that you are taking in only a small "thread" of air. You are trying to take in the same quantity of air you breathe during normal ab breathing, but you want to do it in a small steady stream instead of one large amount.

Quiet refers to both keeping your inhales and exhales silent. Ideally, in thin breathing, you would be breathing so slowly, thinly and quietly, that your abdomen would rise very slowly. An outside observer might not even be able to notice that you are breathing.

I would consider thin breathing as the most valuable practice here for chi development. Having said that though, it's important to work up to thin breathing over a number of practice sessions, by learning the other practices first.

Start by practicing normal breathing first for a few days or weeks, or even a month. Then practice normal ab breathing for a few weeks, followed by reverse ab breathing for a few weeks. Take your time with these practices.

Breathing practices can be done anywhere. Since they are mostly quiet practices, you can even do them when others are around, and most times they won't even notice. They can be done at anytime you have a few minutes to spare.

Once you learn them, you can even combine breathing practices with daily activities, such as sitting in your car in traffic, standing in line at the store, doing the dishes, watching TV, or sitting at the computer.

Anytime during the day when you happen to think of your breathing, do your current practice from the above. Do it while you are thinking of it. Do it even if your attention on your breathing lasts only a few seconds before it goes back to whatever task you are doing. You'll see plenty of benefits (emotional stability, improved health, etc.) by using these practices during your daily life.

Post-Birth *Jing* #3: Chi Cultivation

The third "post-birth *jing*" process is chi cultivation. By "chi cultivation" in this context, we are specifically talking about practices involved in converting the first Treasure "*jing*" into the second Treasure "chi".

Many Tai Chi and Qigong masters consider your ability to convert *jing* to chi efficiently as the most important "post-birth" factor for physical health, emotional well-being, and longevity.

When we talk about the efficiency of *jing*-to-chi conversion, of special concern is the prevention of "*chi dissipation.*" Dissipation refers to the loss of chi during practice.

As an example, think of exercises like running and aerobics. These exercises require us to generate a lot of chi energy. Much of the energy we produce, however, is consumed in accomplishing the task of the exercise, such as running a given distance or performing the aerobics movements for a period of time.

High-level Tai Chi and Qigong require us to generate a lot of energy too — in most styles, just as much as running and aerobics.

But these chi arts have one important distinction. While performing these arts, **we want to conserve as much of the energy we generate as possible,** so that we have an abundance of chi to assimilate and store at the end of our practice.

This assimilation and storage is what gives the chi arts their superior and long lasting health benefits.

I know many of you are just starting on the path to high-level Tai Chi and Qigong. Whether you are a complete beginner, or someone who is experienced in other styles, you should focus your beginning high-level Chi Development practice on preventing chi dissipation and on making your *jing*-to-chi conversion as efficient and effective as possible.

Regulating for Chi Cultivation

When talking about the *jing*-to-chi conversion, Tai Chi and Qigong teachers use the Chinese term *tiao*, which means to "mix, blend, reconcile, adjust, or tune." Specifically in Chi development, we translate the term as "regulate", where it refers to adjusting and tuning our practice to reach a desired goal.

Qigong and Tai Chi involve many levels of regulating, but specifically beginning "Chi Development" students are taught to "regulate" their practice to prevent chi dissipation.

Some of these regulations involve specific structural and energetic alignments, specific types of coordinate movements, specific levels of movement precision, and specific methods of organizing practice sessions.

The Importance of Kinesthetic Details

Given the goal of efficient *jing*-to-chi conversion and preventing chi dissipation, we can't emphasize enough the importance of learning "kinesthetic" details and applying them to your Tai Chi and Qigong practice.

These kinesthetic details include important information about how the movements should feel. These details allow you to feel if you have the proper alignments, coordination, precision, and organization to aid in the *jing*-to-chi conversion.

These types of details are important for every single Qigong or Tai Chi movement you learn. Your teacher or instructional program is responsible for providing this level of detail for every single movement.

So what are these kinesthetic details like? Here's an example, from our description of the exercise *Looking Backward* from Eight Brocades Qigong.

Looking Backward is a simple Qigong pattern that is great for the head, neck, and tops of the shoulders. Many of these areas become frozen or stiff after long hours of sitting, especially at a computer. The simple neck turn of *Looking Backward* can help loosen and relax the muscles, tendons, and vertebrae in the neck and shoulders.

An Example of a Kinesthetic Detail for Looking Backward

Turn from the Lowest Neck Vertebra

In chiropractic terms, the vertebrae in the neck are called the "cervical vertebrae." The highest vertebra, next to your skull, is called C1 (Cervical-1) and the lowest vertebra, near your shoulders, is called C7 (Cervical-7).

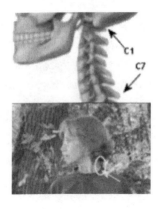

Most people originate their neck turn between C1 and C4 - the upper part of the neck. As much as possible, try to originate the turn from the lower part of your neck (C5 through C7), where your neck meets your shoulders. Turn your neck from the area of the lowest vertebra possible for you.

To do this turn correctly, focus on turning from the neck muscles near the shoulder rather than from the skull. Once again, you may not be able to look backward as far by turning from the lower vertebrae, but it's not how far you turn, it's how well you turn that counts.

Of course, this is just one detail in one movement. Every movement you learn in Tai Chi and Qigong will have several details.

Your instructor - either in-person or through books or videos - must provide this level of detail. (If he or she doesn't provide these details, you are wasting your time learning, you may never achieve real breakthroughs in Chi development, and you may actually be risking injury to yourself through improper instruction. The best advice in this case: Find another instructor!)

The importance of these details is that they allow you to "customize" each and every Tai Chi and Qigong movement you learn. Every movement must be customized in order to prevent chi dissipation, and to make your "*jing*-to-chi" conversions as efficient as possible.

Custom-Fitting for Jing-to-Chi

Let's face it - we all have different bodies, different minds, different energy systems. And if you don't customize the movements to your particular mind/body/chi, if instead you just copy your instructor's movements, your Tai Chi or Qigong will be like one-size-fits-all clothing.

If you are like most people, a "one-size-fits-all" piece of clothing never quite fits correctly. Given that we all have different shapes and sizes, instead of one-size-fits-all, most of us opt for clothing with a range of size options.

And of course, the clothes that will fit you best are ones that you have "custom-made" - cut to your precise measurements, sewn to your specifications, hemmed to just the right size and length.

Well in some ways, Tai Chi and Qigong are just like clothing. Most classes, books, and videos offer a one-size-fits-all approach. You are taught the movements and expected to copy the teacher in a "monkey-see, monkey-do" manner. If you have trouble copying the teacher, well - the only option you have is to practice harder until you can copy the movements and look just like your teacher. After all, in a one-size-fits-all approach, you either do it the teacher's way - or you don't do it!

So as you can see from the example above, even in a simple exercise such as a neck-turn, kinesthetic details allow you to customize the movement. You concentrate on how the movement should feel to you. You pay attention to how you move so that movement is just right for you - not on how well you can copy your instructor's movement.

If you aren't given this level of detail, your Tai Chi or Qigong will be like one-size-fits-all clothing - it will never quite fit you correctly, no matter how hard you practice! However, given the proper kinesthetic instruction, your Tai Chi and Qigong will fit you like a "custom-made" outfit - cut to your precise measurements, made to your specifications, fitted just right for you.

Details like these are designed to help you accomplish *jing*-to-chi conversion easily and effortlessly. Their purpose is to give you all the benefits that Chi Development has to offer.

Eight Ways to Regulate the Body for Chi

In the last chapter, we mentioned the importance of regulating your body during your Tai Chi and Qigong. You want to do your chi exercises in a way that encourages *jing-to-chi* conversion, but conserves as much of the chi as possible.

Consequently, it is important that we minimize *chi dissipation* in order to get the most benefits during our practice. While there are numerous causes of dissipation and numerous solutions depending on which art you practice, there are some universal methods of body regulation common to many chi arts. These methods may help to alleviate dissipation problems and thereby improve our practice.

Method 1: Use Deep Relaxation

One primary cause of chi dissipation is through *tension and the excessive use of strength*. These two factors cause us to use more chi than we need to accomplish the movements of the art, thereby wasting chi.

To prevent this dissipation, most Qigong styles recommend performing movements using deep relaxation.

At a minimum, we emphasize relaxing the muscles deeply so that there is no residual tension during movement.

Beyond this, many arts look to release tension down to the tendons and ligaments that support our muscles, and then even further down to the internal structures, such as bones, bone marrow, and internal organs.

The goal is often to have no superfluous tension at any level in the body - essentially making the body feel transparent and "boneless" during movement.

Through a simple partnered exercise, you can learn to feel this deep level of relaxation during movement.

We'll focus on relaxation in the arms using a simple movement from Tai Chi called *Raise Hands* - though you could substitute any arm movements from your own Qigong form to get the same feeling.

The Raise Hands movement requires you to lift your hands and arms from the sides of your body to in front of your body just short of shoulder height, palms down. You then lower the hands back to the sides of the body.

To experience this movement with deep relaxation, ask two friends or training partners to help you.

Each partner stands along one side of you and takes one of your arms, supporting your wrist and elbow. Both partners slowly lift your arms to shoulder height and then slowly lower them to your sides. Your partners should focus on keeping the movement coordinated, so that your arms rise together always at the same level. In addition, the movements should be performed slowly, taking at least a minute or longer to raise your arms and the same amount of time to lower them.

During the exercise, concentrate on keeping both arms completely relaxed, giving your partners the full weight of your arms. Do not attempt to lift or move them in any way. Your partners should also monitor your arms to see if they feel any change in your level of relaxation or any resistance while both raising and lowering your arms.

This exercise is excellent training for all three of you. For your part, you'll learn to tune in to how it feels to be relaxed completely during the movement. Your partners will learn sensitivity, which is also an essential component in regulating. After several repetitions with their assistance, you should then try to perform the movement unassisted, keeping as close as possible to the same level of relaxation as you had during the exercise.

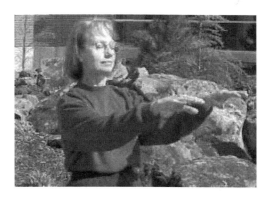

Isolating arm movements from your qigong style is an excellent way to learn body regulation principles such as deep relaxation and gravity-aware movement.

Method 2: Make Your Movements Gravity-Aware

In addition to deep relaxation, learning how to generate movement properly, especially in our arms and legs, can help prevent tension and strength from dissipating our chi.

In the chi arts, limb movement is often generated through awareness of our interaction with gravity. For example, when we want to lift our arms, we need to use just enough force to overcome the pull of gravity. We may refer to this concept, at least figuratively, as using "gravity plus 1 percent."

The goal is to use the bare minimum amount of force to move the arm upward. Using more than this causes us to use more chi than necessary to accomplish the movement. Of course, if the movement must be fast or forceful, you may need to exert more force. However, you should not use more than the amount required by the movement.

To continue the example, when we want to lower arms, we do the opposite. We reduce the amount of force we are using to hold our arms up to less than the pull of gravity. We may reduce it to a metaphorical "gravity minus 1 percent" if we wish to lower our arms slowly, or we may reduce it more than that if we wish to move more quickly or forcefully. Finally, if we wish to be non-moving, we fill our limbs with a force equal to gravity.

Failure to "ride" gravity is a very common cause of tension in chi arts. This habit is a carryover from our daily lives, where we may use much more force than necessary when reaching for objects or opening doors.

To experience this riding of gravity, we may use another partnered exercise similar to the Raise Hands exercise above. This time have just one partner stand in front of you and take both of your wrists in her hands. She should then lift your hands slowly into the air in front of your body, just below shoulder height. Have your partner hold your arms there, while you remain relaxed, giving her the full weight of your arms.

Very slowly - the slower, the better - have her reduce the amount of force she is using to hold up your arms, while you gradually add energy to your arms to compensate.

This should be done over a three to five minute period, while you add only the minimum amount of force you need to adjust for the gradually diminishing support. By the end of the exercise, your partner will have removed her support completely, and you will be supporting your limbs by yourself, with just a small amount of energy.

At this point, slightly reduce the force in your arms. You will find that they gradually and slowly sink downwards. At some point, slightly increase the force and your arms will stop moving. Increase the amount just a little more and your arms will slowly float upwards.

Done properly, this exercise will teach you how to ride gravity during movement, while giving you the feeling of "swimming in air" that Tai Chi and Qigong players often strive for.

Method 3: Use Proper Body Structure

Another common cause of dissipation is improper body structure, such as misalignment of body parts during movement.

Misalignment may cause chi to be locked and blocked in a part of the body or may cause a part of the body to be cut off from chi flow. On a more physical level, misalignment may also cause injury, further exacerbating the loss of chi.

Causes of misalignment are often unique to each person and sometimes may be hard to detect, much less diagnose. Sometimes the misaligned body part is not the real problem, but a symptom of another part that has improper structure.

For example, many Tai Chi and Qigong students have problems with keeping knees properly aligned during "shift-and-turn" type movements.

These movements involve shifting of weight from one leg to another, while simultaneously turning in the same direction as the newly weighted leg.

Many students allow the now-unweighted knee to collapse inward and twist, which may cut off chi circulation to the knees and possibly weaken the knee structure.

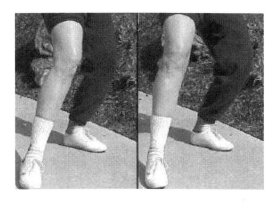

The Qigong student at left demonstrates a common structural problem - twisting the forward knee during a shift-and-turn movement. Structural problems may dissipate chi as well as increase the risk of injury. (Proper alignment is shown at right.)

Unfortunately, there can be numerous reasons why a student may be collapsing his knee. It could be tightness in the inner hip folds (*kua*) and groin, for example. This tightness prevents full turning from the waist, so the student compensates by collapsing the knee in order to increase the radius of the turn. Or the problem could be in the feet or ankles. The student may be flattening the natural arch of the unweighted foot, which causes the ankle and knee to misalign.

In either case, a short-term solution may be to reduce the amount of turn, in order to prevent destabilization of the knee or collapsing of the arch. Longer-term solutions may be to work on flexibility in the inner hips or on strengthening the arch of the foot.

Given the wide variety of possible causes and solutions, it can be difficult to find the exact cause of a misalignment. There is one exercise, however, that can often help. This exercise is called *post standing* in many chi arts.

Method 4: Practice Post Standing

The simplest version of post standing is to take a posture from your Qigong or internal art form and use it for standing meditation.

Hold the posture for at least five minutes and for up to twenty minutes or longer if that amount of time is within your comfort zone.

While holding the posture, try to stay deeply relaxed and to use a minimum amount of force (equal to gravity, as described above) to maintain the pose. Focus on your breathing, on chi circulation, or on any meditation appropriate to your art.

After holding the pose for a time, return to a normal relaxed standing posture, with feet parallel and arms resting comfortably by the sides of the body.

Internally scan your body from head to toe at a slow pace, looking for areas of tension, soreness, aches, excess energy or strength, or places where energy feels blocked or stagnant. Any areas you find may indicate a misalignment during your post standing. After a few moments, return to the posture and hold it again, looking for improper structure either in the areas you identified, or in adjacent body parts that may be causing problems in these areas.

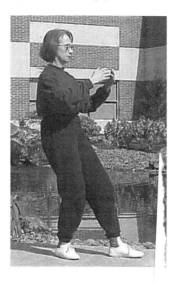

Holding qigong postures for an extend period of time can help you pinpoint problems with tructure and precision during regulatio

You will most likely need to perform post standing ith each posture of your form in order to detect any imprope structures in your practice. This level of detailed practice may seem tedious, but the feedback it provides about your posture is substantial!

If you are new to post standing practices, however, you may want to perform no more than one post posture per day or per practice session, due to the intensity of this practice. This rule-of-thumb prevents overworking your body's energetic systems.

Method 5: Strive for Coordinated Movement

Another possible cause of dissipation is moving parts of the body independently, with no clear linkage to the structure of the body as a whole.

This is very similar to improper structure, but whereas improper structure is often localized and can be seen in static postures, dissipation from non-integrated movement is caused by a more pervasive body misalignment that occurs only while moving.

Independent movement often occurs in the limbs, especially in the arms and hands. Again, this may be a carryover from our daily habits. Especially for those of us who are desk-bound workers, we often move our arms without moving our bodies for long periods of time. Consequently, we may have a difficult time detecting non-integrated movement in our Qigong practice.

However an outside observer, even if they are untrained in our art, is often able to help us detect this problem.

For example, let's say you practice Tai Chi. Since most Tai Chi styles emphasize coordinating arm movements with those of the waist, you can ask a friend or partner to watch you perform a few movements of your form.

Ask them to watch with this one question in mind: *"Do I
·r move my arms prior to moving my waist?"*

ᴄ   ᴄonnected movement will be obvious, even if your
frieɩ ᴊ has never studied Tai Chi.

For the record, we should note that independent movement of parts is not always a defect. As a matter of fact, some forms of Qigong such as *wai dan* ("external elixir") and Buddhist styles encourage it. These styles use localized twisting or bending movements to build chi in one part of the body, such as the limbs, before releasing and redirecting it throughout the rest of the body.

The imagery often used is that of water flowing through a garden hose. As you step on the hose, water stops and builds up pressure, and when you release the pressure, the water spurts through the hose cleaning any blockages.

Likewise, as you twist, you build up chi, which then spurts through the body cleaning any blockages when the twist is released.

Thus in some Qigong styles, independent movement is encouraged and not necessarily problematic. However, many *nei dan* ("internal elixir") and Taoist Qigong styles require complete coordination of the entire body during movement. This coordination is also a prerequisite in most internal martial arts including Tai Chi.

Method 6: Keep Your Form Precise

Many chi arts are designed to activate the body energetically. They may work with certain energy pathways (channels or meridians) or certain energy gates and acupuncture points. Some are designed to work on deeper energetic structures, such as specific organs, the spine, or the bone marrow. Even chi arts that take a more whole-body approach often require a certain amount of precision to achieve the appropriate effects.

Performing a movement or posture incorrectly may reduce the efficiency of the exercise and dissipate chi.

Form imprecision is related to misalignment problems we've already discussed, but here, the practice of regulating requires a more detailed look at our movements.

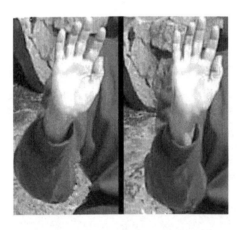

Form precision is often a matter of inches. The "drifting" elbow of the Tai Chi student at left reduces the amount of chi she experiences and impedes this posture's function, which is to express jin (internal force) through the palm. A better elbow position for her style is shown at right.

For example, while a few centimeters difference either way in limb or torso placement may not cause serious misalignment, it may make the difference between success and failure in activating an energy pathway or structure.

Method 7: Be Aware of the Functions of Your Art

Some chi arts have a particular function associated with its movements.

For example, Wild Goose Qigong represents the daily routine and habits of the wild goose, which symbolizes longevity and high energy levels. Other styles may invoke the movements and symbolic qualities of other animals, both real and mythical, such as Constant Bear Qigong. Or they may simulate natural elements, such as Liuhebafa (Six Harmonies, Eight Methods), often called "Water Boxing."

The function is even more apparent in internal martial arts forms like Tai Chi and Bagua, since they involve actual self-defense applications.

To prevent dissipation, it is important to have an understanding of the function of the art.

As one student put it, "your chi needs something to do!"

Without the focus that functional experience provides, dissipation may occur through simple misdirection of chi. Knowing the function and application of each movement of your form prevents this misdirection, and is a critical component of the awareness required to regulate physical movements.

For Qigong players, study the functions behind each movement. Do they represent how a bird builds a nest? Or how fire consumes wood? Or how clouds float through the sky?

For internal martial arts, study the self-defense and *jin* (internal force) applications of each movement. Even if you are interested in only the health benefits of Tai Chi or bagua, being able to express *jin* correctly in martial situations means that the appropriate chi pathways in the body are open and activated.

Method 8: Organize Your Practice

Another way to prevent dissipation is to organize your practice sessions for optimal body regulation and chi cultivation.

Organizing is especially important if you practice a number of chi arts, movement or otherwise, during a single session.

Generally, the routines in the first section of our practice session should encourage deep relaxation; calming the body, mind, and breathing; and opening the chi gates and centers to dissolve any blockages. Much of this preparation section may be given over to non-moving Qigong or to simple single-movement routines.

The preparation section then leads to the cultivation section of our session. Here we are devoted to generating and cultivating chi, as well as developing energy flow. In this section, we may perform our longer, more complicated movement routines or our more challenging non-moving Qigong, such as the post standing described above.

The final storage section of our practice is then devoted to assimilating and storing the chi generated during the previous sections.

Generally this goal is accomplished using non-moving Qigong or meditation. Many arts focus on directing and storing chi in the body's primary energy reservoirs (variously called "channels" or "vessels") and in primary energy centers such as the lower dantien just below the navel. This may be done using guided imagery, breathing, relaxed body posture, or simply the direction of mind-intent.

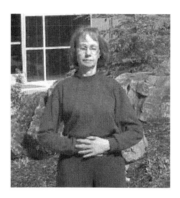

The storage section of a practice session is crucial for chi cultivation and for long-term health. It may involve guided imagery, breathing, relaxed body posture, or simply mind-intent.

No matter how it is accomplished, this final storage of chi is important for our long-term health, as we mentioned earlier.

Unfortunately, we are often tempted to rush through or skip this section in order to get on to the "next thing" in our life.

Skipping this section, though, may mean that we dissipate much of the energy we've just generated, undoing all the good work we've just finished.

Instead, it's better to spend the time saving the energy in our "chi bank account" for a rainy day rather than spending it all on whatever comes next in our life.

Spirit: *Shen* Mind

So far, we've discussed *jing* and chi, two of the Four Treasures. Now let's discuss *shen*, the Third Treasure.

"*Shen*" is often roughly translated as "spirit", but probably "higher awareness" or "personal realization" may be better translations.

However, I prefer an even better translation of "*shen*" as "mindfulness."

Yun Shui – Cloud-Water Mind

When I first started teaching, I called my program "CloudWater Tai Chi. The word "cloudwater" comes from the Chinese word *yun shui*.

This is the word used for the wandering Zen monks so often depicted in Chinese stories and paintings. These monks dedicated their lives to developing mindfulness through practices such as meditation, Qigong, and Tai Chi.

Because of the high level of mental freedom and detachment they developed, they were called *yun shui*. *Yun shui* literally means "cloud-water," referring to a line in a poem that symbolized this freedom as the ability "*to float like clouds, to flow like water.*"

In our courses at CloudWater Tai Chi, *yun shui* symbolizes the personal freedom and enlightenment that can be gained from the Chi Development practices. Some of the practices we teach specifically focus on helping you convert the Chi you develop into *"shen"* or mindfulness.

The mental and emotional freedom of mindfulness complements the physical benefits you'll receive from your practice to create whole body/mind health.

Certain "mindfulness" practices, integrated into your Qigong and Tai Chi exercises, aid you in developing *"yun shui* mind". These mindfulness practices are designed to give you an unprecedented level of freedom in both mind and body.

Shen and Zen Mindfulness

As mindfulness practices, Tai Chi and Qigong have some things in common with Zen, another influence on our practices.

Back in the early 1980's, just prior to beginning Tai Chi, I practiced meditation in general, and Zen meditation in particular, for several years.

Zen is a Japanese discipline that grew out of Chinese Buddhist practices. It's difficult to describe Zen in just a few words, but as one of the first Zen masters said, it is "direct pointing to the real person, seeing into one's nature, and attaining enlightenment."

Both Zen and Tai Chi have a common Chinese ancestry. Taoism, the native philosophy of China, is the mother of both disciplines. For Zen, the father was Buddhist meditation practices, introduced from India into China in 500 B.C.E. For Tai Chi, the parentage was more complex, mixing Taoist meditation and breathing practices with Chinese martial arts and health exercises.

In both offspring, however, we see the influence of the parent's meditation practices. Therefore, it was natural for me, as a student of Zen meditation, to be attracted to a meditative martial art and exercise form like Tai Chi.

As a matter of fact, throughout history, the opposite has also been true: many martial artists have been attracted to the study of Zen.

The samurai of feudal Japan, for example, found that discipline of Zen helped them overcome fear and pride, two of the largest obstacles to effectiveness in combat. But combat effectiveness is not the only reason for studying Zen. Martial artists in all times have turned to Zen to help them become more present in the moment, more mindful, during the practice of their arts.

The most intimate relationship that Tai Chi and Zen have is this connection as mindfulness practices.

Shen and the Monkey Mind

Mindfulness or "*shen*" is the state of mind when we are completely open to the present, aware of what we are doing in this moment. With mindfulness, there are no barriers between us and our actions. We are aware of what we are doing, of the effect we are having on ourselves, on others, and on the world. We are plugged in to the now, without the robotic, emotional programming that normally interferes with our lives.

With mindfulness, we are able to make decisions, based not on the "shoulds" and "oughts" that normally chatter away in our "monkey minds", but based on what is best for the moment. And when we decide to act, we know the action is right because we are aware.

We are not acting from mind, but from no-mind, from a complete identification with what is going on. As such, mindfulness might sound a bit far out, a bit New-Agey-feel-good, or even a bit like a drug-induced trance. It is not. Mindfulness is a practical, down-to-earth state.

It is breaking down the emotionally based habits and reactions, and allowing our true inner nature to shine forth.

To break down this inner programming and develop mindfulness, Zen practice involves seated meditation. Through seated meditation, the Zen student usually focuses on one specific meditative technique, such as counting breaths, chanting, or working on a "Zen puzzle" known as a *koan*. By developing this one-pointed focus, the student will quiet the emotional, robotic parts of the mind and allow mindfulness to emerge.

Some styles of Tai Chi however do not focus directly on mindfulness, or even mention it at all. More attention is usually paid to movement and principles, with mindfulness emerging as a by-product or secondary goal.

However, in higher level Tai Chi and Qigong styles in general, mindfulness is given a primary position. But instead of using the Zen path of "quieting the mind" we use skills developed from the "Three Treasures" to develop mindfulness.

While the lower levels of Tai Chi and Qigong specifically focus on the conversion of *jing* to chi (raw material to energy) and the cultivation of chi, you can view this early work as preparation for the upper levels where *shen* takes a more prominent role.

In the upper levels, we advance to practices that are designed to help with the conversion of chi to *shen* (energy to spirit), to help develop not only radiant physical health, but the mental and emotional freedom of mindfulness.

It's a bit beyond the scope of this book to delve into Zen mindfulness in any great detail. If this is your first encounter with chi-based mindfulness, and you would like to know more, I recommend checking out my first book on the topic of mindfulness, called *Three Monk Mindfulness Volume 1*.

This approach uses chi based practices, along with certain mental and emotional exercises, to help you explore mindfulness. Just go to Amazon.com and search for *Three Monk Mindfulness.*

But for now, let's explore one way of culitivating *shen* through the practice of silent Qigong.

Practicing *Shen* Silence

In the last chapter we discussed cultivating "shen". And one of the way of cultivating "shen" is through the practice of silent Qigong. In this chapter, instructor Jeffry C. Larson talks about the power of practicing silent Qigong.

What does five minutes of silence feel like to you?

I mean real silence. No TV, no radio, no cell phone.

Just . . . silence.

Does it seem empty like something is missing? Do you start to feel bored or maybe anxious?

What if I told you that 5 minutes of silence a day can vastly improve your physical health and mental well-being?

What I am referring to here are the various standing qigong like Embrace the Pearl, Three Circle Qigong, and Universal Post Qigong.

Internal Activity

In each of these exercises there is no external movement. On the outside there should be only stillness. Internally there is a whole lot of activity going on. Lungs are exchanging air, blood is moving, organs are processing, chi is circulating, and the mind is still active.

In fact the reason we cease all external movement in these exercises is to consciously direct our mind to all of these other things going on inside the body. We tend to spend all of our waking hours with our mind scattered across 10,000 things at once. All of us need time in our day to concentrate and shift our focus to the inside.

A Silent Environment

To facilitate this process it helps to be in an environment of external silence, so that you can perceive no activity outside yourself.

However, having said that, I would also say that you could potentially perform these exercises in a variety of places.

You could practice outside in a park where you can feel the wind and hear the birds singing. It's even possible to practice in a crowd of people such as on a train or while waiting in line.

You may have to modify your stance somewhat according to your environment but as long as no one is trying to directly gain your attention you can still direct your mind inwardly.

But if you are just starting out in this practice then seek seclusion as much as possible until you establish a solid foundation of mental focus. Silence is the optimal environment.

Mental Focus

So now that you have established a silent environment and a still body on what do we direct our mental focus?

First, focus on the details of your physical stance for the particular exercise that you are performing.

Pick one detail to focus on, such as your foot placement. Feel your feet from the inside out. Take mental note of how they are aligned. Feel the balance of weight across the entire bottom of each foot. Visualize their rooting into the ground. Take each of the structural details in turn and focus your attention on it.

Take time to focus in on your breathing. Control of your breathing creates a critical link of mind to body. Your cycle of inhale and exhale should be slow and measured. The action of breathing should be centered on your lower abdomen. Feel it expand on the inhale and contract on the exhale. Visualize the air coming into and flowing back out of your body.

Start Slowly

You may find that during prolonged standing that your legs may start to feel "burned-out" and tired. Remember to start slowly. Try starting your standing practice with 1 minute, then each day try to stand just a little bit longer. The key here is a gradual progression.

For this exercise, time is a relative and arbitrary measure. Sure, eventually you want to work up to five consecutive minutes, but there is no set schedule for when you will get there. This practice is for a lifetime, there is no need to rush.

When you begin this practice, even one minute of standing may seem like an eternity. Eventually you will progress to the point where five minutes have gone by with your conscious mind hardly even realizing it.

Keep in mind that when you do start to feel your legs wanting to give out, there is one thing you can do: relax. Take this time to focus your attention and reach out with your mind to really feel your legs from the inside out.

As you do this, you will begin to feel areas of excess tension that are not helping you to stand up. Use your mind to just let those muscles relax. You will be surprised at how much tension you can let go in your legs and still remain upright and stable.

Feel how your body's natural integrity and structure keeps you buoyant without excess tension.

Cultivating *Shen*

All of the standing qigong exercises are about cultivating *shen* mindfulness. With practice you will ingrain this attitude of mindfulness to such a degree that it will carry over to all of your other life activities.

Mindfulness leads to body awareness. You will start to move with more grace and strength in everything you do. Mindfulness centers our consciousness. After practicing these exercises, you will return to activity with calm and focus.

Mindfulness allows our internal energy (chi) to be coherent and heightens our sensitivity to it. You will find yourself better able to fight off "dis-ease" and able to sense illness and injury before they digress into major physical ailments.

I encourage you for the sake of your own physical, mental, and spiritual wellness to find at least five minutes every day to be silent and practice a standing qigong exercise.

I know that our schedules can be so full, some days it can be tough to find the time. Make it fit into your schedule. Any time during the day is fine. Do it daily with the guidelines given above.

If you remain consistent in this practice, you will reap tremendous benefits over time.

- Jeffry C. Larson

Al J. Simon

Check Your Beliefs at the Door

Most Chi Limitations Aren't Physical

Margaret has stroke paralysis. She is wheelchair bound and completely paralyzed on one side. If there were anyone who had an excuse not to practice Tai Chi or Qigong, it would have been Margaret.

But after reading a few of my emails, she wrote me and said, "*Al, I really want to join your online Tai Chi and Qigong program.*"

Well, I was blunt with her, just like I am with everyone. I told her that our students with limited mobility have had mixed success. A few have worked through our online Chi Development course and been very satisfied with their progress. But a few found it difficult, and eventually left the course.

I told her that success really seems to be more up to the person taking the course - their motivation, their goals, their determination, and their attitude - rather than any limitations they have.

She wrote back, "*Don't worry, Al. I have it all figured out. My caretaker is going to help me. Just give me a little time to get my money together, and I'll sign up for the course and take it from there.*"

Well, a few months later, she wrote me back ...

> *"God bless you, Al. I can't thank you enough for this marvelous course. I can do most all the parts of the movements in my wheelchair. I move my good arm, and my caretaker moves my paralyzed arm for me.*
>
> *"I knew you were worried if I could do this. Well, I KNEW this was the right thing, and wanted to do this, and I WILL keep doing it."*

This is just one of many stories I could tell you from the students with health problems or physical disabilities who've been in my courses.

Margaret isn't the only one. We have others in stroke recovery, or with multiple sclerosis, or muscular dystrophy, or in cancer recovery, or with Parkinson's, or with any one of a hundred other serious diseases, illnesses, or physical limitations.

But what this proves to me - and I hope it proves to you - is that most people's limitations in Chi Development aren't physical. They are mental and emotional.

When you have the right mental attitude and the right emotional intent, like Margaret had, almost nothing can stop you in Chi Development.

Unfortunately, I also see many people at the other end of the spectrum. They have no physical barriers to reaching high-level Qi Mastery. Some have been in the peak of physical condition.

But what holds them back are psychological limitations.

Psychological Limitations

For example, I've had accomplished Tai Chi and Qigong instructors - some with decades of experience - join me in my instructor's training program.

In that program are eight evaluations spread over a two year period, where I give them direct and precise feedback about their practice. I will admit that we are demanding in these evaluations.

Now, that doesn't mean these students have to perform these practices perfectly, or be in perfect health, or be perfect in any way. Many of our coaching members have had serious health problems, limitations, and compromises. That is taken into account in our evaluations. So we give them advice customized to their unique circumstances.

But they do have to do the work.

And they do have to work to the highest level they can realistically achieve.

But about 85% of the people who join the instructor certification course do NOT make it past the first evaluation.

They get their first evaluation results, and they are discouraged, especially those who are already teachers. They thought the evaluations would be easy. But when they receive their first evaluation results, they are surprised at how much additional work they needed to do.

Many quit the program after getting their first evaluation. A majority of these people leave the program and never take another evaluation.

It's not because they can't do the exercises. It's not because they can't make the corrections. Many of them are already accomplished practitioners, and many are in good physical shape.

There is nothing physically preventing them from improving their practice.

Instead, what's holding them back tends to be the mental and emotional challenges that accompany the breakthrough to higher level Chi Development.

Chi Development is "Holistic"

One of the greatest Tai Chi masters I ever met in person - whom I'll be mentioning in a moment - once wrote words to the effect that Tai Chi and Qigong needed to be accomplished physically, mentally, and emotionally.

He said the physical part was easy.

The mental and emotional were much harder.

Chi development - at its highest levels - is personally and emotionally challenging.

Any serious changes to your energy system also require changes to your thoughts and emotions.

I would say that's because Chi Development is *holistic*.

Now I don't mean the word "holistic" the way most people use it today to mean "alternative." I mean "holistic" in the original sense of the word.

Your energy system, your physical body, your mind, and your feelings are all tied together.

They are all whole.

So changes to one means changes to them all. You can NOT make serious changes energetically WITHOUT making serious changes mentally and emotionally.

You see, real breakthroughs in Tai Chi and Qigong come about when you free yourself from mental and emotional limitations.

To free yourself, many higher level "secrets" in Chi Development are about changing your mind and emotions to change your energy system, or changing your energy system to change your mind and emotions..

Chi Development and Shen Development

When discussing these types of changes that happen in Tai Chi and Qigong, you may have heard masters use the term *shen* in your Chi development.

As I mentioned earlier , *shen* is often roughly translated as "spirit," but probably "higher awareness" or "personal realization" may be better translations.

However, I prefer to translate *shen* as "mindfulness."

Now before we get too far, "mindfulness" is another one of those words that people today use differently from the way masters of the past used it.

You may have heard from so-called experts and gurus these days that mindfulness is "paying attention" or "being present" or "living in the now" or "being aware" or "dwelling in a non-judgmental state." You may have heard of mindfulness in connection with meditation, breathing exercises, or awareness practices.

But I mean a more "old school" definition of mindfulness. The way we use to define it back when I was a Zen student back in the 1980's, and the way it was defined throughout the centuries.

One of my favorite definitions comes from a 6th century Zen master. He defined it this way:

"Direct pointing to the real person, seeing into one's nature, and attaining enlightenment."

Mindfulness, shen, is about exploring yourself (that is, your "inner self") on a deep level. It's about getting rid of all the programming and robotic thoughts, feelings, and actions that have been layered on top of your personality all these years. It's about finding the real person, the True

Self, underneath that all - the True Self you know you have inside you.

Because that's what Tai Chi and Qigong are about, at their deepest level, at the level of *shen*.

It's about the personal freedom and enlightenment that can be gained from Chi Development.

You see, higher level Chi Development is practically synonymous with *Shen* Development. Chi and *shen* go together at higher levels. It's about taking the energy, the Chi you get from your practice, to help develop not only radiant physical health, but the mental and emotional freedom of mindful shen.

Without this mental and emotional freedom, most students and instructors are limited in their Chi Development. Breakthroughs are hard to come by, if they come at all.

Grounding Yourself

The work we do for *shen* will change the way you think and feel about Tai Chi, Qigong, and Chi development. It will change how you look at and think about yourself and about your place in the universe. It will also change how you think about your students (if you are an instructor), about other people, and even about the world around you.

It will challenge you to get past any robotic reactions, and habitual thoughts and feelings, and help you see, hear, and experience things - both inside and outside of Tai Chi and Qigong - in a new way.

To me, that's some of the highest level energy work you can do.

I realize that if you are new to this type of intense *shen* development, it may be a little difficult to first catch on with what's going on.

So to help ground you in this approach, I have five tips I'd like to share with you.

These are all from Masters from various disciplines. Each of these five tips on mental attitudes can help improve both your chi and *shen* development.

If you can keep these five bits of advice in mind, they will guide you through the emotional and mental challenges you'll be facing as you make your breakthrough to the upper levels of Tai Chi or Qigong.

Better Not Believe

Master Tip #1: "If I believe entirely in books, better not read books; if I rely entirely on teachers, better not have teachers."

This tip is from Master Liang Tung Tsai. Master Liang, who passed away a while back at 103 years of age, was the greatest Tai Chi master I had ever personally met.

During his life, he developed a number of innovations in Tai Chi - new forms, new practices, and new approaches. And that raises the question.

How could such an elderly Chinese gentleman, steeped in formal practice through his studies with traditional masters, become such an innovative maverick of Tai Chi, even into his 80's and 90's?

Master Liang mentions his secret in his book, *T'ai Chi Ch'uan for Health and Self-Defense*. One of his ten "guiding principles" to accomplish Tai Chi mentally warns us, "If I believe entirely in books, better not read books; if I rely entirely on teachers, better not have teachers."

Despite the traditional teaching of the masters he studied with, Master Liang did not stop at solely taking their words, but worked to search out answers for himself.

Some might call this a skeptical, non-believers approach to Tai Chi and Qigong. I have found during my 30 years of practice that this skeptical attitude is something that many high-level Tai Chi and Qigong masters share.

A skeptical approach improves not just your practice of Tai Chi and Qigong, but your ability to develop the mindfulness of *shen*.

Many masters encourage a skeptical attitude in their students. They quite often ask their students to metaphorically "check their beliefs at the door." As a matter of fact, they point out that sometimes a "believing" reaction will impair your development.

These masters encourage you to completely separate what you believe (or disbelieve) from the actual experience of your practice.

You approach your practice time more like a "laboratory research scientist," viewing your practice as a series of "experiments" from which you are gathering results. You focus on gathering results, specifically turning off the parts of your mind given over to interpreting these results.

You should perform your practice not to prove or disprove any theories or principles, but merely to perform certain steps and gather information for - and about - yourself. In this way, you prevent yourself from accidentally introducing "bias" either for or against any results during your practice.

In reality of course, most of us find it difficult to turn off the "belief-producing" part of our mind. But masters using an "experience-based" approach to Chi Development insist on the importance of at least attempting to check our beliefs at the door.

To help us with checking our beliefs, we have our second mental attitude tip.

Empty Your Cup

Master Tip #2: "Empty your cup."

Bruce Lee conjures up the image of a flashy kung-fu movie star, but his personal students describe a more thoughtful, pragmatic teacher who focused on efficiency and practicality in martial arts.

And one of Lee's favorite teaching stories involved the Zen master who likened a student full of beliefs and opinions to a full tea-cup. Before the cup can hold more tea, it must be emptied.

Likewise, without first emptying your mental cup, how can you expect to make any breakthroughs in your practice?

Many times in his writings on the martial arts and self-development, as well as in stories by his students, Bruce Lee taught that we should empty our cup to develop ourselves to our fullest potential.

He was especially critical of practice that consisted merely of rote repetition, principles set in stone, and pat, formulaic answers.

As he once wrote ...

"Formulas can only inhibit freedom, externally dictated prescriptions only squelch creativity and assure mediocrity. Bear in mind that the freedom that accrues from self-knowledge cannot be acquired through strict adherence to a formula."

I find this "breaking away from formulas" to be one of the more difficult mental changes for some Tai Chi or Qigong students - and for many instructors. And I'm not "holier than thou" here. I had trouble breaking away from this myself many years ago.

That's because many of us began our Chi Development with forms - those stylized, choreographed dance movements that most people think of as Tai Chi or Qigong. We learned Tai Chi or Qigong in a follow-the-leader, "monkey-see, monkey-do" fashion, and we begin to think of Tai Chi or Qigong as this pattern of movements. We start thinking of learning movements and forms as the goal, rather than as simply a means to an end.

Plus, and this is even more restricting, we get used to being handed answers by our teachers.

And the truth is, some teachers can be fairly dogmatic.

If a student asks a question, they'll give the student a principle or a practice rule. Or they'll make some sort of correction, or show the student the "proper" way to do the movement.

They'll do all of that rather than do the one thing that would most help the student - and that is to encourage the student to experiment, check their results, and come up with their own answer to the problem.

Breaking out of formulaic thinking and textbook answers is a key way to make breakthroughs in Chi Development - whether you are a beginning student or an experienced master.

And this next tip talks about how to do just that.

Be a Researcher

Master Tip #3: "Be a Tai Chi and Qigong Researcher."

When I met him back in the 1990's, Master Instructor Chris Luth had taught Tai Chi and Qigong full-time for nearly 20 years. He was also a two-time former U.S. National Tai Chi Champion who conducts retreats and workshops around the world.

In 1996, during a retreat in Northern California, I was driving Chris and two other students back from a training session atop a nearby mountain. During the drive, I had asked Chris for advice on a particular teaching problem I was having.

In response, Chris said that when he was confronted with these types of problems, he looked at himself as a "Tai Chi and Qigong researcher." He said that from early on, his Master, Liu Chen Huan, was extremely open-minded, encouraging him to investigate and experiment on his own to find answers and solutions.

So from early in his Tai Chi career, Chris said he looked at himself as a "Chi researcher," and he encouraged his students to do the same thing.

As you may know, I took that advice quite literally, probably even more literally than Chris intended.

It was shortly after receiving that advice that I broke away from my more traditional instructor, and began my own Tai Chi and Qigong program. I started testing everything I taught through student feedback and research. If something worked for my students, I kept in it the program. If it didn't work, we took it out. It didn't matter if it was traditional or if a lot of other teachers did it that way. The results are what counted.

That advice twenty years ago was quite literally the starting point for the successes my students and I have had - and are having still today. This "researcher attitude" is something I pass along to my own students - right from the moment they start training with me.

That's why - right from the start - we encourage our students to customize the practices we teach, so the practices fit them. This is quite different from many Tai Chi and Qigong programs, where you are given movements, practices, and principles, and are expected to copy and reproduce them exactly as your instructor does.

In our courses, we do the opposite. We do NOT want students to copy and reproduce what we do. The students are encouraged to experiment with what we teach, check their results, and at the end, when they've found what works best, adjust their practice accordingly.

I like to say that in our courses, we try to make Tai Chi and Qigong fit the student, rather than make the student fit Tai Chi and Qigong.

Since we say the same thing so often, I started using an acronym for this process.

The acronym was "ECRAA".

The Meaning of "ECRAA"

ECRAA means "experiment, check results, and adjust accordingly."

I remember one time, an "outsider" to our program once asked, "How can students who've taken just a few lessons in your program know enough to make modifications to Tai Chi and Qigong?"

My answer was ...

> "Because we haven't taught them only Tai Chi and Qigong movements. We've taught them a set of skills that includes in-depth body awareness and Chi energy awareness. Even in just a few lessons, they've learned quite a lot about how their body and energy works, and what works best for them.

> Of course, they don't know enough to adapt Tai Chi and Qigong for every person's strengths and weaknesses - after all, that takes more intensive training.

> But even after so few lessons, even the complete beginner will start to know one person's capability intimately - they know themselves!"

As you work your way through more advanced Tai Chi and Qigong, make sure you keep ECRAA in mind. With everything you learn, you should experiment with, check your results, and adjust accordingly.

"Experiment, check results, adjust accordingly" ...

... That's ECRAA.

Of course, to be good at ECRAA, it helps to keep our next mental attitude with you.

Beginner's Mind

Master Tip #4: "In the beginner's mind there are many possibilities, but in the expert's there are few."

This tip comes not from a Tai Chi master, but a Zen master. Shunryo Suzuki-Roshi came to the United States from Japan in 1959, and is often cited as one of the principal founders of Zen in America.

Suzuki-Roshi was not a master of Tai Chi or Qigong, but of Zen. But his advice about "beginner's mind" applies equally well to those of us involved in Chi Development.

Checking our limiting beliefs at the door is one way to keep a "beginner's mind" - full of possibilities during our practice. By focusing on the actual practice we are working on, rather than "expert" theories and principles about Tai Chi and Qigong, we open up to a greater potential for a higher level of skill.

That's the heart of our approach to Tai Chi and Qigong. It's not about principles, forms, or theory. Yes, we do have some theory, but only enough to help you understand the intention of our approach and our practices.

Instead, we want you to "experience" Chi Development, not just think about it. We want you to have these experiences in a "personal" way, unclouded by "external" theories of what you are supposed to experience or what is supposed to happen.

Speaking of beginner's mind, we have another saying in Chi Development that's very similar:

"One man's master is another man's beginner"

If you've been around Tai Chi or Qigong for any length of time, you've heard this saying.

Of course, as with most clichés, it's literally true. Being a master of one style, or one program of Chi Development, does not necessarily give you an advantage in other styles or programs.

Actually, sometimes previous learning is a limitation, even a hindrance. You might find that you have to "un-learn" things that you've learned elsewhere. You may have to open your mind to new things you are learning, especially when they contradict what other teachers may have told you.

But despite its literal truth - the saying is also about attitude. It's about being willing to let go of past learning, and giving yourself over to new processes.

Beginners Mind in Action

Here's one of the best examples of beginner's mind I ever personally witnessed.

In 1985, I attended a week long martial arts training camp. This wasn't in Tai Chi or Qigong or in Chi work, but in a martial art that focused exclusively on self-defense and combat. This was the annual training camp for this style, and about 400 people or so had come from all around the world to train.

Much of the training in this style was two-person or multi-person. So in the workshops during the camp, we'd be shown certain techniques and then practice them with a partner or group of partners. Generally at these camps, you tried to pair up with people you didn't know. It was a good way to get a lot of experience with many different training partners in a short time.

At this one particular workshop, we were about to do the partner training. The person standing next to me asked me if we could work together.

Now, this guy looked familiar to me, but I didn't recall having met him before. He introduced himself as Tom. He was a small Asian fellow. I was about a foot taller than him, weighed more than him, and since I was in my 20's, I was probably 10 or 15 years younger than him. Maybe more, I'm not a good judge of age.

But he had amazing skills. It was clear right from the start that he was new to the style we practiced, but he was picking up all these techniques quickly. The whole time I'm working with him, I'm thinking, "I've seen this guy before," but I couldn't place where.

As we continued to work on the techniques, I threw in a variation I had learned previously from my personal teacher back home. He said, "*That was very good. Could you show that to me?*"

Well, just as I was showing him, the master of our style, who had organized the entire week-long event, walked over and said to Tom, "*Master so-and-so, no one told me you were here. It's an honor to have you with us.*"

And as soon as our master said that, I knew who my training partner was. This guy was a well-known master in another style of martial arts. He was in a number of martial arts magazines I read back then. As a matter of fact, I had read one of his articles on his style just a few weeks before. And he wasn't just a master of his style. He was the highest ranking master currently living in the United States for that style.

In fact, between this guy and the master of our style, I had standing in front of me the two highest ranking people in the United States in each of their respective martial arts.

Anyway, the master of our style said, "*Master so-and-so, we would be pleased if you would join us for a demonstration, or to teach some of your art. Is that something we could work out with you during this week? Or at least could we introduce you to our students here?*"

And this master said, "*Oh, no, thank you very much, but I'm sorry, not this week. I'm just a student here. And please stop with the Master so-and-so. Just call me Tom. I'm really just here to learn. My friend Al here has already taught me something new.*"

That episode had a big impression on me, as a young martial arts student. Here was a well-known master, a guy with decades of experience, who was literally putting "beginner's mind" into practice, right before my eyes.

While I've forgotten many of the techniques I learned at that camp over 30 years ago, I remember Tom and his beginner's mind clearly.

And that leads us to our final mental attitude ...

Initiative

Master Tip #5: Don't wait for it. Take the initiative.

While all of these tips have come from other masters, this is my own master's tip for this list.

Because initiative is really what helped me reach where I am today. It's really the key secret that led me directly to becoming recognized as a Qi master and inducted into the U.S. Martial Arts Hall of Fame.

I've had initiative all along during my career in both the martial arts and the Chi energy arts, and it has carried me far.

Here's one example. One of my early Tai Chi instructors taught a variation of the Yang 108 movement form. Now, it really wasn't Chi development. It was what I now call "monkey-see, monkey-do" choreography, but that's all I knew at the time. But even at that level, it took about six months for the class to really learn the 108 movements.

Now, we finished just before a four week break before the classes resumed. At that last class before the break, the instructor said that when we came back, we would start relearning the 108 movements, but in the reverse direction, mirror-imaged.

Well, during the four-week break, I worked my tail off teaching myself the mirror-imaged version of all 108 movements. I still had a full time, corporate job back then, but I spent at least two hours every morning and one to two hours every evening to get it done. I learned the whole thing on my own.

When we came back, I waited until the end of the first class, and asked the instructor if I could show him something.

I then performed the entire 108-reverse that he had just begun teaching.

He asked me how I learned it, or if I had already known it, since he knew I had taken Tai Chi before studying with him. I explained what I had done. He made about a dozen corrections, then asked me to become his senior student.

That eventually led to private lessons with him and my first Tai Chi teaching assignment.

I have a second story that is also similar. It happened about 10 years before the last story though.

In another martial art - the combat art I talked about earlier - we had a group that met on Wednesdays in a park and on Fridays in a studio.

On one Wednesday evening in the park, the instructor was late, which had never happened before. When he didn't show after about 10 minutes, I suggested to everyone we get started, and I started leading the class through the warm-up exercises.

Keep in mind, I had only been training in this style for seven months. I'm just a white belt in a class of white belts, and I'm the least experienced person there. Some of the other students had been training for almost a year. (Now, this particular style had very few belt colors, and long periods of time in each belt grade. Usually you spent at least a year as a white belt.)

Well, we were almost finished with the 20 minutes of warm-up exercises, when we saw the instructor walking across the park. When he got to where we were, everybody stopped, and I said, *"I'm sorry, we started without you. Hope that was OK."*

He looked at me a little oddly, but said, *"Just fine. Why don't you keep going?"* and had me finish leading the warm-ups.

Six weeks later, he awarded me the next belt color, without testing, and with only about nine months as white belt. He said, *"When I walked into the park that night, and saw you had not only taken the initiative to start, but that everyone there had followed you, I knew you were ready to be a green belt."*

And that opened the doors for me for more training and experiences.

The Single Biggest Skill

So I'm not telling these stories to pat myself on the back. They were so long ago, they don't really matter.

But they point to the fact that the single biggest skill that will take you where you want to go in Tai Chi, Qigong, and Chi Development is initiative.

Someone with strong initiative but average Chi skills will achieve a lot more than someone with great Chi skills but no initiative.

But of course, if you do have that initiative, your Chi skills won't stay "average" for long.

Don't wait around for someone to "hand it to you".

No matter what your goals are for your Chi development - just for your own basic health and well-being, or to reach out and teach others, or even for higher levels of *shen* development for psycho-spiritual achievement - you need to make the choice and commitment to go after what you want for yourself.

And you need to give yourself over to the process.

Make the commitment right now to take the initiative and follow through on what you've started here.

The Tao of Change

Ask just about anyone why they became involved in Tai Chi and Qigong, and they will tell you that it was because they wanted "something better" for themselves.

Whether it is improved health, stress relief, exercise, martial arts, personal development, or just about any other reason - the reasons most of us became involved in the Chi arts was a desire for improvement at some level.

As a matter of fact, wanting something better is the reason we do most things in life.

It's why we exercise, why we diet, why we choose a career or change jobs, why we develop relationships - just about everything.

But most times, the changes we need to make in ourselves to pursue what we want are difficult.

It's why most Tai Chi and Qigong classes and programs have a drop-out rate between 40% to 80%, according to various studies.

It's why most diets have an even higher drop-out rate. It's why so many people make New Year's resolutions in January that are completely forgotten by March.

Let's face it - change is difficult, even if the change is for something we want.

How many times have you wanted to practice Tai Chi and Qigong more? To eat a better diet? To get a new job, or to have better relationships? And how many times have you started off with good intentions, but faltered along the way especially when the changes required became difficult?

So what if there was a way to make these changes easier?

The Taoist Path of Motivation

Tao Jia just might have an answer for you. *Tao Jia,* translated in English as "Taoism" (but pronounced "Dow-ism"), is one of several philosophical systems from China that have influenced Tai Chi and Qigong. And one of the most important contributions of Tao Jia is the concept of *wei wu wei.*

Wei wu wei literally means "do/not do" or "act/not act". Sometimes you may have seen this phrase shortened to *wu wei* ("not-do") and translated as "inactivity".

But in Taoism, *wei wu wei* does not mean doing nothing at all. Rather, it is "doing something" so effortlessly that it appears easy. It represents a way of pure effectiveness and effortlessness action, so that you become so totally focused on the action, that outside distractions and roadblocks disappear.

Wei wu wei, effortless action, holds the key to making change easier. When we become so totally focused on our actions, what we are doing becomes effortless, and reaching our goals becomes easy.

So how do we reach effortless action?

"Unify Your Attention - Listen With Chi"

To reach effortless action, the *Tao Jia* philosopher Chuang-tzu tells us:

> *"Unify your attention. Rather than listen with the ear, listen with the heart. Rather than listen with the heart, listen with the chi."*

Here he points that the way to "effortless action" is through chi development. Chi is truly the "Taoist power" that drives the "Tao of Change."

It has been said that *wei wu wei* is the pinnacle of *shen* mindfulness development. Our actions become effortless when we are able to direct our chi to help us make change easier and are able to accomplish our goals. A person who has developed "mindfulness" is one who can set and reach goals for themselves.

But it's not just ancient texts that say that. Even modern psychologists have noticed the intimate connection between "reaching our goals" and "developing chi."

Dr. Lee Milteer, who has a Ph.D. in Motivational Theory, puts it this way: *"All energy creates results. Take charge of your life energy, using the mental, physical, spiritual and emotional energy to your best advantage."*

An important component of Chi Development is "focused intention."

Focused intention is what makes your *"wei"* (actions) appear *"wu wei"* (effortless).

By focused intention, what we mean is having a clear idea of what you want (intention) and having the necessary mental awareness (focus) on the actions that will achieve our intention.

In simpler terms, to create real *shen* mindfulness change that brings us something better, whether in Tai Chi and Qigong, or in "real life", we need three things - (1) intention, (2) action, and (3) focus.

Of these three, **intention is generally the easiest** for most people. Most of us have things we want. To practice Tai Chi more regularly, to lose weight, to get a better job or career, to have better relationships, to be happier, you name it - we all have things we want.

So "intention" is usually not where we falter. **Where we usually falter is in "action" or in "focus."**

For example, many people want to improve their health, but few actually begin the necessary dieting, exercise, or lifestyle changes to reach their goal. They've faltered at the "action" step, failing to do what needs to be done.

But even those that begin dieting or exercising often fail to keep with their diet or exercise plan. The vast majority quit after a few weeks or months. They've faltered at the "focus" step, failing to provide Chuang-tzu's "unifying attention" on the actions to reach their goals.

It would be tempting to say that these people simply lacked "willpower" or "commitment". But it's not that simple.

The truth is that many of us today are just not "programmed for success" in Tai Chi, Qigong, or life!

We know how to have the desire/intention, but we've never learn basic motivation skills such as how to overcome roadblocks and past failures; how to eliminate catastrophic thinking; how to refuse to be a slave to circumstances; how to seize opportunities when they are presented; how to develop creative problem-solving; or how to capitalize on past success to produce present success.

But these skills in "intention - action - focus" can be learned. And to see these skills in action, I'd like to explore two examples from my personal experience.

The *Wei Wu Wei* of Teaching Tai Chi

The most effective, "effortless" Tai Chi classes and self-study methods make "intention - action - focus" explicit in the teaching.

The instructor shows the students how the "actions" they are learning relate to their "intentions", then provide the "focus" on what part of the "actions" accomplish those intentions.

For example, the lessons in our programs and courses strongly emphasize "intention - action - focus."

Every lesson starts with the "intention" of the skill being taught - why you are learning the skill; how it will affect you physically, mentally, or energetically; what benefits you can expect from the skill.

Then we follow it up with "action" - a step-by-step lesson plan of how to perform the skill. This "action plan" is specific, with detailed information on how to perform the skill.

Finally, we follow up with the action plan with "focus" - specific steps to pay attention to in the action which will guarantee that you fully realize the intentions/goals of the action.

Good instructors provide these important motivations. Poor ones don't.

I knew in my own teaching I had "turned the corner" on this skill when our dropout rate in our in-person classes went from about 70% to under 10%. We stopped accepting new students, as our classes would start full, and stay full. Capturing a student's interest, and keeping them coming back for more, became effortless on our part.

Developing a Tai Chi Career

Of course, in the "real world", most of us don't have "instructors" that keep us on the "intention - action - focus" path. Instead, in the real world, we need to learn on our own or from others the motivational practices that will keep us going towards our goals.

I too had to learn these practices in a "real world" situation nearly twenty years ago.

At that time, I was laid off from my high-paying job when the high-tech company I worked for went out of business. By the time I was laid off, I had grown dissatisfied with my limited options working for corporations. I wanted more career freedom to explore all the areas I was interested in, such as Tai Chi and Qigong, developing educational courses, and helping people with "service-oriented" technology. And as most people do, I wanted greater financial independence.

I knew that I wanted to create a new future for myself as a Tai Chi and Qigong teacher, writer, and publisher, especially in the new (at that time) world wide web.

Like most people, I had the "intention" - the easy part - but the action part was another matter. My fears and doubts held me back - after all, this was after the "tech bubble" burst in the early 2000's, after 9-11, and while the country was in a recession. I had very little money in the bank, I was facing an uncertain financial future, and most of all, I was afraid to change.

Removing the Roadblocks to Success

But of course, I had to remove a number personal roadblocks to "action" and "focus". To remove these roadblocks, I had help. I spent time learning techniques to overcome difficult situations and circumstances; to learn to take chances; and to capitalize success. I spent time "programming" myself for success using the power of intention, action, and focus.

As Dr. Milteer puts it, *"By redefining your thoughts and actions, you unleash (almost by magic) your true creative potential and achieve a spirit of excellence."*

No matter what you want out of life, you can begin to use the "Taoist Chi" power of *"intention - action - focus"* in your own life.

You'll soon see yourself changing for the better and realizing your goals, whether it's to improve your Tai Chi and Qigong practice, to improve your health or diet, a better career, better relationships ... just about anything.

And you'll make the changes effortlessly (*wei wu wei*), bringing you a high-level of success you might only be able to imagine.

Power: Internal *Jin*

Now that we've explored essence *(jing)*, energy *(chi)*, and spirit *(shen)*, it's time to turn our attention to *jin*, the Fourth Treasure.

Earlier in this book, I mentioned that *jin* is often translated "internal power" or "intrinsic energy".

In its widest possible definition, it refers to the outward expression of our cultivation of *chi* and *shen* to the world around us.

In martial arts and Tai Chi, *jin* often narrowly refers to the expression of chi to generate power in movement.

In more spiritually-oriented disciplines, *jin* may refer to how we use our "higher awareness" to reach even higher levels in our path to the highest level of "personal enlightenment" or "emptiness."

Usefulness

One of the main ideas behind these definitions of *jin* is "usefulness" - using chi to accomplish a particular goal. **And that is actually an excellent definition of *jin* - using chi to accomplish a particular goal.**

The goal here can be something physical (such as generating power in movement) as well as something non-physical (such as "higher awareness").

When it comes to the non-physical, we've actually already covered much of what is involved with *jin* in the previous chapters on *shen*. And specifically, the last chapter about *wei wu wei* is all about "non-physical jin" - using your chi development to reach a particular goal.

Since we've covered the non-physical, let's turn our attention to the more physical definition of *jin* usually used in Tai Chi - using chi to generate power in movement for a specific purpose or goal.

This definition has two important parts: (1) using chi to generate power in movement, and (2) using the movement for a specific purpose.

Generating Power

Using chi to generate power is actually the easiest part of learning *jin*.

Let me give you a simple example.

I have a little experiment I do when I teach Tai Chi called *Pushing the Wall*. It's a little trick I use to get new students to FEEL what Tai Ch should feel like. It's a simple to do, and it may even be something you tried as a child. But it will give you a good feeling of what *jin*-generated power feels like.

Here's the experiment you can try for yourself.

Do the following movements slowly.

1.   Stand in a comfortable stance with some distance between your feet. Your arms should be at your sides, with your elbows turned out slightly.

2.   Inhale and lift up your arms slowly, until your hands are somewhere between chest and shoulder height.

3.   Exhale and lower your arms slowly to your sides, back to the way they were in Step 1.

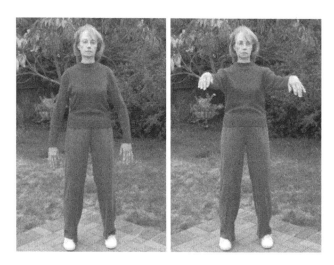

Repeat this "lifting arm" movement a few times so that you get the hang of it before continuing.

Now Try This Experiment

Now here's the experiment you can use to feel the "gap" between movement and awareness.

Important Note:

If you have any health concerns, you might want to take it easy with this Pushing the Wall experiment. Especially if this is your first time doing anything like this, respect your body's limits and don't overdo it. And if you have hand, arm, shoulder, neck, or back problems, you may wish to NOT do the exercise at all.

But if you are relatively healthy, GO FOR IT!

If you decide to try this exercise, make sure you follow these directions precisely. If you don't, you won't get the proper feeling that we want you to experience.

1. For this experiment, first perform the "lifting arm" movement you learned above about 5 to 10 times. Pay special attention to how your arms feel each time you lift them into the air.

2. Now you will need to stand facing a sturdy, blank wall. Stand as close to the wall as possible, and place the backs of your wrists against the wall.

3. Now, push as hard as possible against the wall with the back of your wrists. You should push VERY HARD! The harder, the better. Use every bit of strength you have to push against the wall with your wrists. You should push harder and harder for about 10 to 15 seconds.

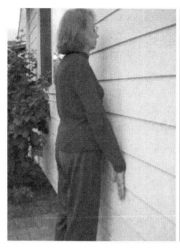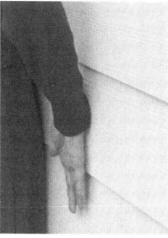

4. Now take a 5 second break, then push against the wall a second time. PUSH REALLY HARD! Push even harder this time, for 10 to 15 more seconds. The harder you can push, the more successful this experiment will be. Push, push, push, and push more!

5. Now take another 5 second break, then begin pushing again. If your arms are getting tired, don't stop! We want to push as hard as you can for 20 to 30 seconds this time. KEEP PUSHING AND PUSHING - DON'T STOP! The harder you push, the better this experiment will work. Keep pushing, keep pushing.

6. After about 20 to 30 seconds, step away from the wall. Now perform the original "lifting arm" movement again, paying attention to how your arms feel. Does the movement feel differently this time? Try to describe to yourself the difference

between how your arms felt in step 1 above, and how they feel now.

Experiencing *Jin*

If you performed the Pushing the Wall experiment and followed our directions precisely, your second set of "lifting arm" movements should feel quite differently than your first set did.

Your arms will feel more like they are "floating" or "rising" by themselves. The movement will feel more effortless and relaxed.

Once they have done the experiment, most students tell me:

"Wow! It feels like my arms are floating by themselves! So this is what Tai Chi should feel like!"

Yes, that really is what all Tai Chi movements should feel like. But all we've done with this exercise is get the muscles we have conscious control of out of the way, and let muscles we aren't normally aware of do the work.

From this little experiment, you've actually gotten your first experience of using chi to generate movement

The experiment shows you how "relaxed movement" and "deeper layer muscles" can be used to allow chi-generated or chi-propelled movement. This experiment is easy to learn, and works almost instantly, despite the fact that some Tai Chi students take years (or decades) to learn relaxed movement. So in this simple, little experiment, you get a brief experience of *jin* using our usual process-oriented approach.

So that's the first part of our "physical" definition of *jin* - using chi to generate power in movement. But the second part actually more difficult - using movement for a specific purpose.

That's where the concept of "intention" really comes into play.

We used "intention" in our previous chapter on *shen* to mean "wanting or desiring something". But in physical Tai Chi "jin", we mean something a little different.

In Tai Chi, "intention" signifies "understanding the purpose of a given movement and expressing that purpose as you perform the movement."

Intentional *Jin*

Every movement in Tai Chi has many levels of "intention" or "purposes" - health, stress relief, Chi cultivation, martial applications, etc.

But when looking at the "intention" of movements in Tai Chi, we often refer to the martial applications of the movements in our discussions.

As you may know, the movements of Tai Chi come directly from Chinese kung fu. And as such, it's sometimes easier to determine the *jin* involved by looking at the martial application of the movement.

However, the intentions aren't limited to martial applications. The intentions have direct influence on our health, stress relief, Chi cultivation, etc. It's just that it's often easier to understand, see, feel, and explore the *jin* by referring to the martial intention.

However, the martial intention can be used to help identify the other intentions as well.

When it comes to *jin*, Tai Chi masters have identified over 50 different "intentions" for generating power through chi. Many of these *jin* are extremely specialized, and it has been said that it is impossible for anyone to master the entire list. Indeed, most Tai Chi masters specialize in just a handful in their practice and their teaching.

However, most agree that there are eight important intentions on the entire list, and that every Tai Chi student should at least be familiar with these eight.

They are the so-called "Eight *Jin*" or "Eight Energies" of Tai Chi you may have heard about. They are:

1. Peng jin ("Ward-off energy")

2. Lu jin ("Rollback energy")

3. Ji jin ("Press energy")

4. An jin ("Push energy")

5. Cai jin ("Pluck energy")

6. Lie jin ("Split energy")

7. Zhou jin ("Elbow energy")

8. Kao jin ("Shoulder energy")

We will discuss these Eight Jin in a later chapter. But before we do, we need to take a more in-depth look at the role of intention Tai Chi. We also need to be able to spot Tai Chi intentions in our practice.

It will take us the next several chapters to cover Tai Chi intention, but it will be time well-spent. When we return to the Eight *Jin* in a later chapter, you'll see how these chapters on Tai Chi intention greatly simplify our task of understanding the Eight *Jin*.

Tai Chi Intentions

The Role of "Intention" in Tai Chi

Thousands of years ago, our ancestors observed the natural processes they found in the world around them.

As part of their observations, they began classifying the fundamental "building blocks" or "elements" of these processes.

Many of these original elements - air, fire, water, and earth - wouldn't be called elements in today's science. But they do represent the fundamental building blocks of the world as the ancients experienced it in their time.

As serious Chi researchers, we also seek out the fundamental building blocks of our "Tai Chi universe." And just like those ancient thinkers, we too will use the elements of air, fire, water, and earth to help us understand these fundamentals.

Our search for the fundamental elements of Tai Chi begins by looking at the role of "intention" in Tai Chi.

By "intention," we mean specifically that every Tai Chi movement you learn has an intended effect, and you should "express" that intention as you perform the movement.

What makes Tai Chi so complex to learn, yet so powerful to practice, is that every pattern of movement in Tai Chi actually has multiple intended effects. '

Multiple Intentions

These multiple effects arise from the fact that Tai Chi combines a number of practices into a "holistic" system. In one complete system, you get:

- physical exercises originally derived from martial arts, plus

- energy work derived from Qigong, along with

- breathing and mental concentration derived from meditation.

Instead of having to practice physical exercises, energy work, and meditation separately, you can practice them all together and increase the benefits you get exponentially.

Of course, if you just learn the physical movements of Tai Chi as you do in most classes, books, and videos, you will only learn a small part of the system. And unfortunately that means you only get a small part of the benefits!

So to get the maximum amount of benefits, it's important that you learn about all the effects - physical, martial, energetic, and mental - that Tai Chi is trying to create in your body and mind. The best way to ensure you get these effects is to create them "intentionally." By intentionally producing the correct effects, you will do more than just increase the benefits you get. You'll also decrease the amount of time it takes to learn, and your practice will become more meaningful and more enjoyable.

Because Tai Chi combines the physical, the energetic, the martial, and the mental, you may think there is an overwhelming amount of "intentions" to learn for each movement.

However that's not the case.

The Principles for Intentions

We can simplify the learning process with three simple principles, and still get a large amount of benefits from our practice.

1. **We can select and focus on just a single "primary" intention in each Tai Chi movement.**

Tai Chi movements often have multiple effects on all levels. But we can often select one of these intentions as the "primary effect" to create for the movement.

If you focus on the primary intention, often times the secondary intentions will "fall in line" and produce themselves automatically.

So if you learn a primary intention for each movement, and focus on learning how to express that intention with your body and mind, you'll often get the full range of health, energy, and stress relief benefits from Tai Chi.

2. **The multiple aspects in a given Tai Chi movement generally work together towards the primary intention.**

Instead of viewing each aspect of Tai Chi - the physical, mental, martial, and energetic - as having distinct intentions, most Tai Chi movements use all of the aspects to express the same primary intention.

For example, we might select "expansion" as the primary purpose for a given Tai Chi movement. If "expansion" is indeed the primary intention, the movement then usually expresses "expansion" physically, mentally, martially, and energetically. Working on "expansion" in this movement covers all of these areas.

About Martial Intentions

Even though the movements of Tai Chi come directly from Chinese kung fu, the idea of martial arts in Tai Chi seems to rub some people the wrong way.

We often get email from Tai Chi students and teachers who say they aren't interested in martial arts, and that they only practice for their physical health, mental peace of mind, and/or spiritual well-being.

As you may have guessed, we aren't concerned with whether you practice Tai Chi for martial arts or not. As always, your practice should be customized to your personal goals.

So if you practice just for health and well-being, learning about martial intentions – even if you don't practice them – is still relevant to your goals.

Seeing how the same intention expresses itself in all aspects - physically, mentally, martially, and energetically - will increase your knowledge and understanding of that intention.

Even if you do not practice the martial application of the intention, you will still understand and be able to express the intention better if you've looked at it in all its aspects.

And the better you can express the intention, the better the results you'll have physically, mentally, and energetically - and at any other levels you pursue in your personal practice.

3. **We've identified four primary intentions in just about every Tai Chi movement.**

To make learning the intention in Tai Chi movements even easier, we've identified just four primary intentions that beginning students should focus on.

Just about every movement in Tai Chi expresses at least one of these four as its "primary" intention.

So as you learn each movement in Tai Chi, you can speed up your learning process by focusing on which of these four intentions the movement expresses.

Armed with these three principles, you'll find that your practice becomes more meaningful, more enjoyable, and more results-filled.

Learning Tai Chi becomes more than copying movements as if they were "dance choreography."

Instead, it becomes the key to creating results for your physical health, mental well-being, energetic wholeness, and just for the joy of playing with movement and energy.

Four Elements, Four Intentions

As we mentioned in the last chapter, we've identified four primary intentions that students should focus on in their Tai Chi movements.

To make the four intentions easy to learn and remember, we've "mapped" these four intentions to the "Four Elements" of *air, fire, water,* and *earth.*

This Four Element mapping is drawn from the traditions of both Eastern and Western mysticism. Ancient philosophical and mystical writings from Greek, Indian, Chinese, and Japanese cultures feature variations of the Four Element theory we will be using.

You can look at the Four Elements, and think of them as "metaphors" or "imagery" to help guide you in learning the intentions.

In addition, the elements can be seen as "short-cuts" to discussing Tai Chi intention, since it is much easier to say the word "Air" than to say "the intention of expanding outward, filling, and rising."

And by remembering "a balloon inflating with air" (the Air element) during a movement, it may be easier for you to create the effect you are intending rather than having to focus on concepts that are less tangible.

Let's take a look at, think about, and get a feel for each of these Four Elements and how they apply to our Tai Chi practice.

Air: Rising and Expanding

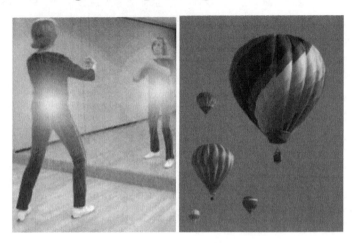

Imagine for the moment a hot air balloon filling with air, then rising into the sky. Or think of the airbag in a car opening and inflating. Or visualize blowing up an inflatable mattress with an air pump. All of these images depict the rising, filling, and expanding nature of Air.

Air movements in Tai Chi involve some sort of expansion and/or rising intention.

You may be physically moving in such a way as to expand outwards or upwards, usually with your arms. Energetically, you may be trying to "fill" your entire body with chi, inflating yourself like an "energy balloon". Martially, you may be creating a protective "air shield" around you, like an airbag that protects a car's occupants.

Each of these elements has many benefits, but let's touch on just a few for Air movements.

Physically, these movements are said to expand the blood vessels and open up space around the internal organs in the body cavity.

Mentally and emotionally, they help us develop a protective "space" to help us feel calm, relaxed, and untouched by stress, fear, or negative emotions.

Energetically, Air movements help increase the *Wei Chi* field, the "energy shield" that acts as a protective layer outside our body.

Spiritually, Air represents our "higher" intellectual functions, our ability to speak, plus our noble ideals and aspirations. Air movements tap into our "expansive" abilities by improving our mental powers, our ability to express ourselves, and our dedication to making ourselves better people and the world around us a better place to live.

As you can see, all of these components - the physical, mental, emotional, martial, and spiritual - show us the rising, expanding, and filling nature of Air in Tai Chi.

Fire: Intensity and Directness

Have you ever felt the intense heat from an open flame? Or have you ever seen how a forest fire spreads quickly and directly, overwhelming everything in its path? Or have you ever watched a flaming arrow shot from a bow, flying directly toward its target? If so, you've seen and felt the intensity and directness of Fire.

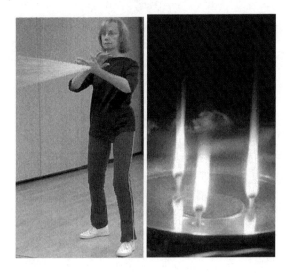

Fire patterns in Tai Chi involve directness and intensity.

Physically, you may be moving in a straight line, or moving along the most efficient and direct path possible. You may be energetically trying to send your energy away from you in a straight line.

Mentally, Fire also symbolizes assertion, not in the form of anger or aggression, but in acting with intense focus and concentration.

Fire movements have many benefits. Physically, Fire movements are said to improve arterial circulation - the sending of oxygenated blood from the heart to the organs and extremities. Fire movements also help us to concentrate on our joint alignment, especially in our arms.

Mentally and emotionally, these movements develop concentration and focus to achieve our goals at all levels. Energetically, the movements help send chi energy along the meridians in our body out to our limbs.

Spiritually, Fire represents our passion, dedication, concentration, and love in all forms. Focusing on Fire helps us improve our passion and commitment to personal goals, plus helps us express our Higher Self/Higher Power in more personal ways to our friends and family.

Whether you practice Tai Chi for physical, emotional, martial, or spiritual purposes, the Fire movements help you develop intensity, directness, and focus.

Water: Retreating and Gathering

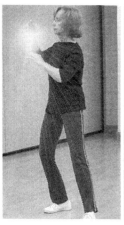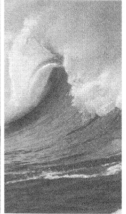

Imagine a vast ocean of rolling waves, each wave gathering, cresting, crashing forward, and then rolling back for the next wave. Or think about the patterns of tides on the beach, as the tide comes in and goes out, coming forward and then retreating. Especially focus on how the waves pull back, retreat, and gather momentum for the next crest.

These images show us the retreating and gathering nature of Water.

Water patterns in Tai Chi involve rolling back and gathering. Physically, you may be moving backwards or pulling your arms toward you. In some Water movements, your arms may actually imitate the cresting of a wave, as the instructor demonstrates in the photo above.

Energetically, you will be gathering energy into you, often times directing it to your *lower dantien* energy collector. Martially, you will be retreating and protecting yourself, as well as gathering and collecting yourself to continue.

Among their many physical benefits, Water movements are said to improve venous circulation - the return of blood to the heart for re-oxygenation. These movements also allow us to work on spinal and joint mobility.

Mentally and emotionally, Water movements help us soften internal resistance and increase sensitivity to what is going on around us. On an energy level, Water movements help us pull chi energy from outside ourselves and our extremities into our internal organs to nourish them.

Spiritually, Water represents our compassion both for ourselves, our family and friends, and to people, places, and things in the world around us. Water also represents security, safety, peace, and tranquility.

In Tai Chi, whether we look at the physical, energetic, emotional, or martial, Water provides us with compassion, security, safety, and peace of mind.

Earth: Stability and Grounding

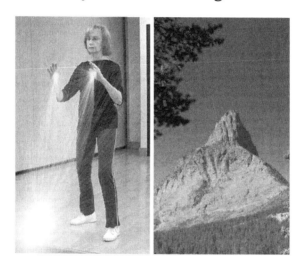

Have you ever seen a large mountain? Both the size and age of these mountains call to mind stability and endurance. Or have you ever tried to push a large rock or boulder just with your arms? Often boulders are impossible to move, due to their massive weight. Both mountains and boulders are images of stability and solidity of the Earth element.

Earth patterns in Tai Chi involve stability and grounding. Physically, you may not be moving at all, or moving only slightly. In addition, you will most likely be pushing downwards towards the earth with the movement.

Energetically, you will be sinking your energy into the ground, making yourself energetically heavy. Martially, you will be holding your ground even during the most difficult situations.

Physically, Earth movements are said to contract blood vessels, keeping our circulatory system active and strong. Earth movements also allow us to work on joint alignment in the legs for a solid connection to the ground.

Mentally and emotionally, Earth movements allow us to deeply relax into stability, allowing us to "hold our ground" even during the most stressful situations. Energetically, we will be focusing on our connection to the ground.

Spiritually, the Earth represents those characteristics that make us human. As such, the Earth center represents grounding and stability, and becomes the ultimate symbol of our humanity

Whether our goals in Tai Chi are spiritual, emotional, martial, or physical, Earth movements allow us to explore stability and solidity in dealing with the world around us.

Spirit/Void: The Fifth "Non-Element"

Now that we've looked at the Four Elements in Tai Chi, we should say something about a "fifth component" you'll find in the Four Element mapping we use.

This fifth component we call Spirit or Void.

Technically, the fifth component of Spirit or Void is not an element, which is why we call this a "Four Element" mapping rather than a "Five Element" mapping.

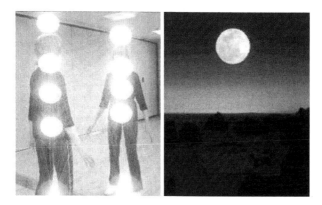

The Spirit/Void, instead of being an element, symbolizes a "coming together" of all the elements into a whole. In this way, it is more of a "non-element" or a "super-element", having a different purpose from the other four elements.

To understand the Void "non-element", go outside at night and take a look at the vastness of space as seen in the night sky. Even in a night full of stars, notice that there is much empty space between each star. The universe encompasses everything, yet is mostly made up of a void of empty space.

Likewise the Void "non-element" in Four Element theory comprises all of the elements, creatively mixed and interplayed. The Void represents our ability to freely use the elements of air, fire, water, and earth to open our minds and body, and to enlighten our Spirit.

Spiritually, it allows us to tap into our Higher Power/Higher Self to draw energy from the universe around us. Focusing on the Spirit/Void center helps us feel more connected to our Higher Selves and to the world around us.

Your "Guide" to Tai Chi

Now that you've been introduced to the Four Elements - Air, Fire, Water, and Earth - plus the fifth "non-element" of Spirit/Void, you may be wondering, *"How will this help me in learn about intention in Tai Chi? What benefits does understanding these Four Elements provide?"*

As you'll soon see, this Four Element mapping comprises a complete physical, energetic, martial, and spiritual guide to learning Tai Chi.

These elements will be your guide to learning the "primary" intention in each Tai Chi movement. You'll discover how the same intention expresses itself in all aspects - physically, mentally, martially, and energetically. This information will increase your knowledge and understanding of that intention.

Armed with this information about the four primary intentions, and about the way to express them in your Tai Chi, you'll find that you'll greatly increase the benefits you get. The Four Elements become the keys to creating results for your physical health, mental well-being, and energetic wholeness.

And by intentionally producing the correct element in each Tai Chi movement, you will do more than just increase the benefits you get. You'll also decrease the amount of time it takes to learn, and your practice will become more meaningful and more enjoyable.

With the Four Elements, learning Tai Chi becomes more than copying movements as if they were "dance choreography." Instead, the Four Elements will turn your Tai Chi from a static, lifeless "copycat" practice into a dynamic, flowing, invigorating part of your life.

Four Elements or Five Elements?

Some of you may be aware of a "Five Element" theory popular in books on Tai Chi, Qigong, and Traditional Chinese medicine.

Now that you are familiar with our Four Element mapping, you may be confused as to the difference between our Four Element mapping and this other Five Element theory.

Those familiar with Chinese Five Element theory may have noticed that it has three of the same elements as our Four Element mapping - Fire, Water, and Earth.

However, Five Element theory does not have either the Air element or a Spirit non-element that we have in the Four Elements. Instead, Five Element theory has Wood and Metal elements.

Realize that whether you are using Four Element theory or Five Element theory, you are simply using a "mapping" of concepts and ideas onto a set of elements.

The elements in and of themselves are not "real," but merely handy devices for understanding a set of concepts or ideas.

As we've said, these elements are used as "mappings" of concepts onto elements. As such, neither the Four Element map nor the Five Element map is "true" or "false" or "the right one" or the "wrong one."

As an analogy, think about maps of a physical location, such as a city. For example, you can have two city maps - one that shows the streets in the city, and another that shows a geological survey of the same city.

Neither map is "right" or "wrong." It's just that one is more or less useful in any situation. If you are driving a car, the street map is more useful. If you are looking for earthquake fault lines, the geological map is more useful.

To extend this analogy, trying to drive using a geological map would be difficult, if not impossible. So keep in mind that Four Elements and Five Elements are different maps, and you need to use the right map at the right time.

For learning about intention in Tai Chi, we've found the Four Element map more useful than the Chinese Five Element map. That doesn't mean that Five Element theory is wrong; it's just not as useful for our purposes. So for the rest of this book, we will use Four Element theory, because for our purposes in learning intention.

The Yin and Yang of the Four Elements

As we delve further into the Four Elements in upcoming chapters, you will learn that these elements are based on the concept of yin and yang in Tai Chi.

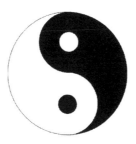

I would guess that nearly everyone reading this book has heard of yin and yang, or at least seen the yin-yang symbol shown here.

But how many students really understand what yin and yang mean - not in vague terms - but in concrete, practical terms both inside and outside of Tai Chi?

For example, I once received an email from a Tai Chi student. He was asking about the principles of "yin and yang" in the practice of Tai Chi:

Dear Mr. Simon,

From some reading materials I was informed that in Tai Chi, "if left leg is yang then right arm will be also yang; if left leg is yin then right arm will be yin." For some Tai Chi postures I comprehend perfectly, but other postures do not fit this principle. What is your explanation?

Thank you,
James

Yin/Yang Is Misunderstood - Even Among Chinese

As Chinese Tai Chi Master Wong Kiew Kit has said ...

"Yin-yang is probably the most widely used Chinese concept in the English language; it is also one of the most misunderstood - even among Chinese!"

So it's no wonder that there is a lot of confusion surrounding these terms.

To understand yin and yang, we need to first look at the origins of these concepts.

Many people are unaware that the terms "yin" and "yang" originally came from the observation of sunlight and shadows.

The ancient Chinese noticed how the sun would shine on one side of an object illuminating it, and how the opposite side would be darkened by shadows.

They also noticed that there wasn't a clear demarcation between the "sunny" side and the "dark" side, but variations of light changing to darkness as you walked around the object.

They also noticed that as the sun moved across the sky, the patterns of sunlight and shadow would change, demonstrating an "ebb-and-flow" nature to the experience.

From this initial "visual" experience of light and dark, the Chinese eventually noticed similar ebb-and-flow in other sensory experiences - sound (with degrees from loud to soft), touch (from hard to soft), sensation (warm to cold), and kinesthesia (motion to rest).

They also began detecting ebb-and-flow patterns in other experiences, such as time, weather, seasonal changes, cycles in nature, our health, cycles of birth and death, cycles of work, and many more.

All of these experiences that strongly excited or stimulated the senses, such as sunlight, loudness, and motion, the ancient Chinese called *yang*.

When the senses were stimulated weakly or not at all, such as in darkness, quietness, and rest, they called it *yin*.

However, the ancient Chinese realized the yin and yang are not "absolutes", but descriptions of the ebb-and-flow in sensory experiences.

They did not think of yin and yang as "forces" or "polar opposites" or "principles" as many people call them.

Instead, they used yin and yang as a way of categorizing and describing ebb-and-flow within a given experience.

In modern terms, we would call categorizing and describing in this manner a "mapping" of experiences onto concepts.

And as with all mappings, the Chinese pointed out that calling something "yin" or "yang" can only be done relatively - in relation to a given experience.

To decide that something is "yin" or "yang" (or anywhere in between) is to select certain characteristics and emphasize their importance, while ignoring or downgrading other characteristics.

Yin and Yang "in the Street"

As an example of this "relativity" of yin and yang, let's pick a simple, everyday object, such as a street light pole like the one pictured here.

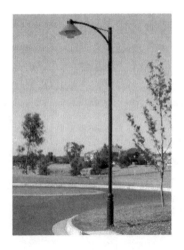

Is a street light pole yin or yang or something in between?

Think about it for a moment ...

The answer of course is that a street light pole can be either yin or yang or anywhere in between, depending on which part of our experience we choose to emphasize.

For example, the pole gives light. So compared to objects that don't give light, the pole falls closer to the yang (sensation stimulating) end of the visual experience.

However, compared to the noisy motors of cars that may pass it, the street light pole is more quiet, so it's more yin (mild to no sensation) in the auditory experience.

But by walking up to the pole and putting your hand on it, you might notice that it is essentially hard, so to the touch, it seems more yang.

However, since you can walk around it and it doesn't move, to our sense of motion it is more yin.

We could continue on, finding a number of both yin and yang characteristics, depending on which part of our experience of the light pole we choose to emphasize.

Tai Chi wasn't Originally Tai Chi

How do yin and yang apply to Tai Chi?

Well first of all, you may be surprised to learn that the term "Tai Chi" originally did not refer to movement exercises or martial arts.

Instead the term was first used to refer to this relative mapping of "yin" and "yang".

Yes, the term "Tai Chi" for many, many centuries referred to the ebb-and-flow of yin and yang.

Though the exercises you now know as "Tai Chi" have been around for three or four centuries, it is only within the last half of that time period that they've been called "Tai Chi".

How did these movements acquire this name?

A Chinese scholar by the name of Ong Tong, after watching a demonstration of the movement art in the 1800's, said that the movements seemed to be a physical manifestation of "Tai Chi", the ebb-and-flow principle of yin and yang.

Hence, the movement art eventually came to be called "Tai Chi", the same name as the ebb-and-flow experience. (For clarity's sake, I refer to the movement art as "Tai Chi" and to the mapping of ebb-and-flow as "yin and yang".)

The Yin and Yang of Learning Tai Chi

Though we call the art after this ebb-and-flow principle, the role that yin and yang plays in teaching Tai Chi varies widely among instructors.

Despite this wide variation, we can simplify our discussion of yin and yang in Tai Chi instruction by exploring the role it plays in three different instructional methods.

Generally, we can categorize Tai Chi instructional methods into three types, giving each type a name that begins with the letter "E" to make them easier to remember.

So let's look at the role of yin and yang in each of the three primary methods that instructors use.

Yin and Yang in the "Exercise" Method

Teachers who use the "Exercise" method of instruction primarily teach Tai Chi and Qigong as movements to be learned and practiced.

Students are expected to learn and, with practice, be able to duplicate the movements shown to them. Student accomplishment is measured by the number of movements or sets (groups of movements) they can perform.

If an Exercise method instructor mentions yin and yang while teaching, they usually do so to help the student better learn the movements being taught.

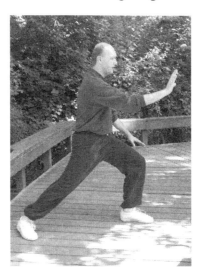

For example, they may use the yin-yang concept to help the students remember and focus on how weight is distributed between their feet in certain Tai Chi movements.

In the movement shown above, an Exercise instructor would point out that since the player is carrying most of his weight on his left leg in this movement, the left leg would be called "yang". The more passive, right leg would then be called "yin".

As another example, the instructor might focus on the position of the hands within the movement. In the movement, the right hand is more forward and extended than the right. The leading, right hand would be called "yang", while the left hand in its supporting role would be called "yin". Using the terms "yin" and "yang" then becomes a "verbal shorthand" for the Exercise teacher to help the students learn and remember which leg or hand is "taking the lead" in the movement.

Unfortunately, we've found that real benefits for health, stress relief, and vitality often take quite some time using the Exercise method. Students often have to learn and memorize a large number of movements before they see tangible benefits.

So while yin and yang in the Exercise method may help you learn more movements more quickly, it won't necessarily improve the level of benefits in your practice. That's because "more" in Tai Chi and Qigong does not always translate to "better".

Yin and Yang in the "Explanation" Method

Teachers who use the "Explanation" method of instruction primarily teach Tai Chi and Qigong as sets of principles to be explained, understood, and demonstrated.

Movements are taught, but students are expected to learn not just movements, but the principles behind the movements as the teacher explains them.

Student accomplishment is measured by the number of principles they are able to either verbalize or demonstrate in their movements.

If an Explanation method instructor mentions yin and yang while teaching, they too might introduce the concepts in the same way as an Exercise instructor.

They might first mention that the concepts refer to "weight distribution" in the legs and/or to "leading" or "extending" movements with the hands. They might also mention "yin" and "yang" in other body parts during Tai Chi, or in other practices as well.

But Explanation instructors often continue on from this point to establish general principles of how yin and yang should be "used" or "demonstrated" in the movements.

They might talk about the "balance" of yin and yang you should have in your movements, or whether your movements should be more "yin" or more "yang", or how yin and yang should be "distributed" throughout your body.

An excellent example of this type of teaching is given in the email at the beginning of this article. James had read that "if left leg is yang then right arm will be also yang; if left leg is yin then right arm will be yin." Even though the email doesn't mention who made this statement, we can easily identify it as coming from an Explanation method instructor.

Especially in terms of yin and yang, we've found two major problems with the Explanation method principles like the one just stated.

First of all, the principles that this method establishes about yin and yang are often treated as 100%, iron-clad rules. And that "fixed", dogmatic mind-set of the Explanation method is at odds with the ebb-and-flow nature of yin and yang in "real-life" Tai Chi movements.

For example, the principle James mentions - that weight distribution and hand position should be coordinated so that the opposite hand and leg are yang - is quite commonly mentioned by Explanation method instructors.

In this principle, if your left leg is forward or has the most weight, then your right hand should be the one that is forward.

However, there are dozens and dozens of Tai Chi movements that violate this supposed iron-clad "yin/yang" principle.

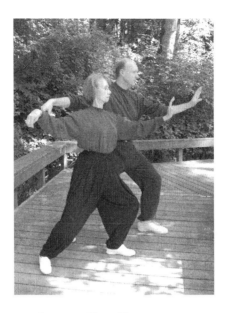

One of the most famous Tai Chi movements, shown here, is called "Single Whip" - and it has both the same hand and leg forward.

Now I've heard these exceptions "explained away" by Explanation method instructors in many different ways. But I would say that most of the explanations are not satisfying, for several reasons:

Sometimes, through some sort of intellectualization, they "explain" that the forward hand "really isn't" yang even when it is forward, and that more focus should be put on the hand that isn't forward. However, this explanation ignores the essential bare fact of how these movements feel when done - that is, they feel like same-side leg and arm should have most of the focus.

Often times, the Explanation instructor promoting this "opposites" principle fails to account for the energetic and martial intentions of the movements. These intentions sometimes require that "yang" or "yin" be in the same-side leg and arm for specific energetic and martial purposes.

Finally, these instructors fail to realize there can't be iron-clad rules or dogmatic principles about a process that is supposed to ebb-and-flow.

Instead, our practice should encompass the ebb-and-flow of all experiences within Tai Chi, whether it violates a "principle" or not.

Beyond this dogmatic approach to principles, the second and more important problem with the Explanation method is that being able to "verbalize" principles and/or "demonstrate" them in your movements does not mean that your internal experience is identical to someone else who also "verbalizes" and "demonstrates" the same principles.

Hence, results in health, stress relief, and chi experiences may not be consistent from student to student. This method may also give students a "false" sense of understanding.

It's false in the sense that real Tai Chi and Qigong breakthroughs, especially in Chi experiences, are related to increased internal awareness and sensitivity, not to verbalization or demonstration of principles.

Yin and Yang in the "Experience" Method

Teachers who use the "Experience" method of instruction primarily teach Tai Chi and Qigong as a series of "experiences" to go through and/or "experiments" to try.

Movements and principles may be taught, but students are expected to perform personal experiments to check the results - positive or negative - of these principles and movements.

Student accomplishment is measured by their attempts at the experiences and their personal results. Teachers of this method work to ensure that the students don't just outwardly mimic the teacher, but that the movements "feel" the same way to the students as they do to the teacher.

Ironically, an Experience method instructor may hardly ever mention yin and yang. These instructors often bypass all the "verbalizing" and "intellectualizing" about yin and yang, and give you practices that will move you to a direct, immediate experience of yin and yang.

The experiences and practices they give you will embody ("put into your body") and "em-mind" (put into your mind) the ebb-and-flow that is a hallmark of Tai Chi.

Experience method instructors will provide you with many different ways to experience ebb-and-flow through movements and energy awareness. They may do this subtly in some movements or more directly in other movements. Some movements may even be taught using the yin-yang symbol as a guide

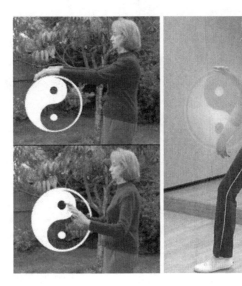

In this way, you learn how the movements actually follow the ebb-and-flow depicted in the yin-yang symbol. With this approach, you'll learn some of the most important physical embodiments of yin-yang in Tai Chi.

Experiencing Yin and Yang

As you may have already guessed, from this chapter and from other parts of this book, I am strongly biased towards the Experienced method of instruction.

As a matter of fact, the not-so-covert purpose of this book is to help students and instructors move away from the Exercise mindset ("Tai Chi and Qigong as movement") and from the Explanation mindset ("Tai Chi and Qigong as principles."). Instead, I'm trying to help them move more towards and Experience mindset, turning movements and theories into experiments and experiences.

As such, sometimes I find answering "simple" Tai Chi questions can be difficult. Not because the questions are difficult, but because the questions are often asked from one mindset – say the Exercise or Explanation mind-set – but really need to be answered from the Experience mind-set.

For example, I'm often asked "What style of Tai Chi do you teach?" That question quite often comes from the Exercise mind-set - that is, Tai Chi taught as movements. And nearly as often, I'm asked to "explain" a Tai Chi principle, which comes from the Explanation mind-set.

So these simple questions are not so simple.

To answer the question, I need to spend time "breaking the mindset" of the question so that we can increase the level of understanding between us.

Without this understanding, my answer might be misinterpreted as an "Exercise" or "Explanation" type answer - which would take us farther from our goals of understanding rather than closer.

So as far as yin and yang, I can now answer the question James posed. James asked:

> From some reading materials, I was informed that in Tai Chi, "if left leg is yang then right arm will be also yang; if left leg is yin then right arm will be yin." For some Tai Chi postures I comprehend perfectly, but other postures do not fit this principle. What is your explanation?

My answer is that in the Experience method of learning, we don't concentrate on "yin" and "yang" as absolutes. They are always "relative" concepts or mappings.

As such, we don't develop rules or principles about yin and yang. Iron-clad rules and principles about yin and yang are seen as contrary to the ebb-and-flow nature of yin and yang!

They tend to limit our experiences, rather than open us to a wide variety of experiences.

The Yin and Yang of Experience

Instead, we focus on ebb-and-flow as experiences.

Yes, you will develop "principles" in the Experience method, but they will be seen more as "rules of thumb" or approximations of the experience, not iron-clad rules. We might say that "mostly" or "many times" or "some of the time" when the left leg is yang, the right arm is yang.

But we would also to be quick to point out that something like that isn't always true. Sometimes our practice leads us to different experiences. So we would never try to enforce such an observation as a rule to be observed during practice.

In other words, "experience" is always in the driver seat. The experience determines the principles, instead of the principles limiting the experience.

So with experience in the "driver seat" of your Tai Chi and Qigong, you'll find many combinations of "yin" and "yang" outside the "limitations" imposed upon you by Exercise and Explanation methods of learning. If you follow the the Experience mindset diligently, you'll eventually learn to open up and feel ebb-and-flow (and apply it correctly) in your practice, and not be limited by iron-clad rules about what is a "correct" experience.

This "opening up" is why so many accomplished Tai Chi and Qigong students and instructors switch over to the Experience method at a certain point in their development.

This mindset opens you up to a wider variety of experiences, and allows you to take the experiences and skills you'll learn, and apply them to a wide variety of learning situations.

Being adaptable, creative, and self-sufficient is what distinguishes Experience method students and instructors from those in more run-of-the-mill Tai Chi and Qigong programs.

So What Do the Masters Say About This?

So you may wonder, how do classical Tai Chi masters look at this Experience approach to yin and yang?

I think no one summed it up better than the greatest Tai Chi master I had ever personally met, GrandMaster T. T. Liang, who passed away at 103 years of age.

One of his students tells this story. During a two-person exercise, one of Liang's most senior students began pushing with his right hand while he had weight on his right foot, making both of them "yang". Though he was in a better position in the exercise than his partner, he remember the principle that yang should not be in the same-side hand and foot, and stopped pushing.

Liang looked at the student and asked, *"Why did you stop?"*

His student replied, *"I can't. If I push from this position, I will be violating one of the Tai Chi principles you told me about!"*

Liang shook his head and laughed. *"So what,"* GrandMaster Liang said. *"If it works, use it!"*

The Inner Warrior

How would you react if someone physically attacked you right this minute? What would you do if, without warning, someone punched at you or grabbed you right now?

What would be your "natural" reaction in that situation? What would you do, almost without thinking?

If you have any training in the martial arts, I want you to forget about all of your training for a moment. What would you do if you weren't trained?

Would you step back out of fear? Or would you strike back in anger? Would you attempt to push away your attacker? Or would you be stubborn and hold your ground?

Which would you do "naturally" - without thought, without hesitation, and without training?

Martial Arts Without Chi

Back in 1984, when I started my training, the usual path to learning self-defense was through hard/external martial arts, such as karate, judo, and jiujutsu, with taekwondo just starting to become popular.

However, my introduction to martial arts training at that time was different. Though I later went on to study some of the "hard/external" martial arts, my first years were spent in the soft/internal arts. I trained in Tai Chi first, and then moved on to other complimentary arts that practice applications that involved the "Four Chi Elements" approach that we discussed earlier.

Since my introduction to the martial arts was through Chi Development, I was actually a bit surprised the first time I stepped into a hard/external martial arts class.

In these hard classes, students were training to overcome fear, anger, surprise, and all the "normal" reactions to sudden physical confrontation.

Through the use of repetitive two-person drills and free sparring, the students were working to acquire and develop "more effective emotional responses" (as some teachers may have phrased it). Students were expected to learn to let go of fear and anger, and instead feel calm, relaxed, confident, and competent in self-defense situations.

There's much to be said for this type of training, and for the ability to feel calm, relaxed, and confident when physically attacked.

But those of us who've ever been in a physical conflict know that ultimately emotions such as fear, surprise, and anger are normal reactions.

Students who've trained long and hard in the training hall may find these emotions taking over if they encounter physical conflict "in the street."

Unfortunately, most martial arts instructors - and this includes a vast majority of the "Tai Chi as martial arts" instructors - fail to train students on what to do when these emotions take over.

With the goal of producing the serene, competent, confident "warrior", few programs address how to defend yourself when you are completely afraid, or thoroughly angry, or even just completely overwhelmed.

Working With Your Body, Not Against It

When I first began in Tai Chi and in the soft martial arts, our goal was not to replace these natural reactions to physical conflict.

Instead, we spent a majority of our applications work exploring these instinctive, natural reactions, and learning how to use them in self-defense situations.

Maybe I was tainted because of my early introduction to Tai Chi and the "energy-based" martial arts, but I always missed this "fighting-how-you-feel" approach when I trained in the harder arts. That is why I never stuck with the hard-style arts for very long, and always returned to Tai Chi and the Four Elements training.

In this style of training, and as always in Chi Development, the approach is to work <u>with</u> your body and mind, and <u>not</u> against them.

Instead, Chi Development tells us that it is not fear, or anger, or surprise that causes us to be ineffective in a physical conflict. Instead, it is our resistance to these emotions that causes problems.

The goal of Chi Development is not to replace these emotional instincts, but to learn to make our actions reflect what we naturally and instinctively want to do.

For example, your natural reactions to being attacked might include backing away from the attack, turning or twisting your body away from it, or even "gathering into yourself" by pulling your arms closer to your body to protect yourself.

In many martial arts, these "fear" reactions are undesirable, and the goal of training is to learn to remove and replace them.

But in Tai Chi, these natural body motions are actually incorporated into the training.

Even on as simplistic a level as forms practice, you'll find these types of motions occurring over and over.

As one example, in just the first 17 movements of the 108-movement Yang Long Tai Chi set, you'll find these "fear reaction" movements are worked into the form nearly a dozen times.

Becoming an Inner Warrior

When it comes to martial arts training in Tai Chi, most students and instructors think about topics such as *jin* (power), *fa-jin* (expressive/explosive power), *dim-mak* (pressure point strikes), and how to apply the strikes, kicks, punches, and throws that are shown in the Tai Chi forms.

For Chi Development students though, these "techniques" come second. Instead, students first work on getting their "head" out of the way of their "body", so that they can naturally express the full force of their instincts and emotions in conflict.

Thus when I first learned techniques like pressure point strikes, we always trained by looking for which strikes worked better when fear takes over, which worked better when anger takes over, which work better when I wanted to hold my ground, and which worked better when I want to maintain control and/or distance from my attacker.

In this way, the techniques would be easier to remember and apply in stressful situations, and would fall naturally out of whatever I felt at the time.

So before you can train in specific martial techniques, you first need to know yourself well. You need to explore which reactions are natural to you, and how to use those reactions to your advantage at all times.

And while we've been talking about this in a martial arts sense, this understanding of natural reactions applies not only to physical conflict, but non-physical interactions with others, and even conflicts within ourselves.

Once you've explored these reactions within yourself and others, you are truly on your path to becoming an "inner warrior".

Al J. Simon

Tai Chi's Natural Reactions

For most people, their first classes in Tai Chi consist of learning choreographed series of movements, called "sets" or "forms". These sets have anywhere from 24 to 150 movements (depending on the style you learn) that the student must memorize and perform in a precise order.

If the student has a good teacher, after learning the choreographed set of movements, she will begin exploring the "skills" behind the movements. She will work on separate drills and practices to learn these skills.

Once she has the skills down, she will then work on how to incorporate these skills into the sets and forms she already knows.

That's how I was introduced to Tai Chi - and how many of you were too.

However, this is the reverse of the way Tai Chi was traditionally taught.

If you go back and read the stories of the original masters of the 1800's and early 1900's, you'll see that their training was quite different. Often, they spent their early years on single postures, single movements, and skill-based drills, before ever learning to connect the movements and drills into sets or forms.

A number of masters claim that this traditional method builds skill much more quickly than the "forms-first" backwards method taught today. When we were developing our courses, we tried both approaches, and our research and student feedback supported this approach. Students saw benefits much more quickly if we worked on skills first, and sets later in the program.

Spotting Natural Reactions

As I mentioned in the last chapter, the practices of Tai Chi, including Tai Chi sets, are built around a set of "natural reactions" to conflict situations.

Note: This is also true for some, but not necessarily all, Qigong forms. To make this discussion more easy to follow, we'll stick with Tai Chi here, since the examples of natural reactions are more obvious in Tai Chi. But keep this in mind if you also practice other movement-based Qigong forms.

One way to apply this understanding is to look at your current Tai Chi and Qigong forms, and to see if you can spot these "natural reactions" in them.

Earlier, we mentioned "The Four Elements", and we describe the intentions behind each of these elements. We'll base our exploration of these natural reactions on these elements.

Complexity of Tai Chi Reactions

What makes Tai Chi so complex is that we often mix and match these natural reactions rather freely. This mix-and-match approach occurs throughout most Tai Chi sets, usually in short sequences, and even sometimes within a single movement.

But when you first integrate Four Elements skills into your existing forms, I recommend forgetting about the complexity.

Instead, find a primary or predominant reaction in the movement, and focus your intention on that Element.

This will help you build skill more quickly than if you try to focus on all the reactions, or on trying to switch quickly between reactions. Often times, you'll find the secondary intentions fall into place of their own accord if you focus on the primary intention.

To help us find and focus on these primary reactions, we often refer to the martial arts applications of Tai Chi movements. As you may know, the movements of Tai Chi come directly from Chinese *kung fu*. And as such, it's sometimes easier to determine the natural reaction involved by looking at the martial application.

However, the natural reactions aren't limited to martial applications. The natural reactions have direct influence on our health, stress relief, and Chi Development.

For example, did you know that each of the natural reactions are said to have a different influence on your cardio-vascular system?

One of the four reactions specifically focuses on arterial circulation - the sending of oxygenated blood from the heart to the organs and extremities. Another of the four focuses on venous circulation - the return of blood to the heart for re-oxygenation. And the other two focus on creating certain effects on the blood vessels.

And of course, that's just the cardio-vascular system. For each natural reaction, you can find effects on certain internal organs, on certain structural elements (joints, bones, ligaments, tendons, muscles), and of course on one of your most important organs, the brain. Each natural reaction also has specific mental/emotional/spiritual effects. The multiple levels of effects of these natural reactions are what make Tai Chi valuable for health, stress relief, and Chi development.

Let's look at an example of each of the Four Elements/Natural Reactions.

Earth Reactions

Yin/yang: Greater yin.

Images: Mountains; large rocks.

Physical reactions: Holding ground; dropping or sinking; pushing or directing downward; compressing; adding weight/heaviness.

Emotional reactions: Miserable; sad; bored; tired; stable; grounded; grounding; immovable; heavy; contracted.

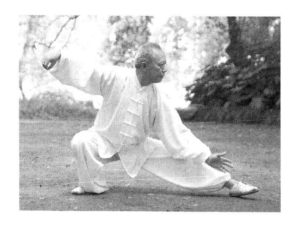

Earth reactions generally involve holding ground, sinking, and/or dropping. If footwork is involved, it will generally be done "in place" with no retreating. If there is any stepping, it tends to be only a small step.

The movement shown here is *Snake Creeps Down*, also known as *Squatting Single Whip*. It is a classic example of an Earth reaction. From a standing position, the player sinks downward.

On a health level, Earth reactions tend to focus on the legs. You'll work on both muscular development and joint alignment in the legs in order to keep a solid, connection to the ground. You will generally find some type of folding or sinking in the legs, usually by bending the knee and hip joints. This is especially challenging when the weight is mostly on one leg.

While not all Earth movements have the extreme squat seen in *Snake Creeps Down*, at a minimum the limbs of the upper body will either be moving downward, or held steady but pushing down. On an emotional level, Earth movements relieve stress by exerting a downward, calming influence on the brain and entire nervous system.

Water Reactions

Yin/yang: Lesser yin.

Images: Tide going out; waves gathering and cresting.

Physical reactions: Retreating backwards; turning sideways; pulling inward; protecting yourself.

Emotional reactions: Alarmed; angry; afraid; annoyed; frustrated; sensitive; empathetic; compassionate; softening.

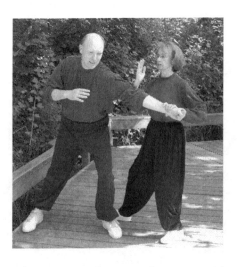

Water reactions generally involve retreating, turning sideways, and/or pulling inward.

Generally, you will be shifting your weight backwards or away from the situation in front of you. If footwork is involved, it will usually involve stepping backwards or pulling your free leg and foot in toward your support leg. The arms usually pull in towards the body. In many Water movements, one of your arms may actually imitate water in the form of an ocean wave that rolls back, crests, and then crashes forward.

On a health level, Water reactions allow us to focus on spinal and joint mobility. The sideways torso movements allow us to take our spine and hips through a greater range of motion, while the "wave crest" movements allow us to work on the shoulder joints.

Water movements relieve stress by softening internal physical resistance, allowing the nervous system to relax, increasing sensitivity, and providing a sense of security.

In the photo above, you see the player on the right performing a Tai Chi movement known as *Rollback*.

You see a number of classic Water reactions in this movement. She is shifting backward and turning away from the attack in front of her. Her left arm is pulling backward, off-balancing her opponent. Finally, her right arm is just about to turn over as if it were a wave cresting, to put pressure on her opponent's elbow as she turns.

Fire Reactions

Yin/yang: Lesser yang.

Images: Open flame; a flaming arrow.

Physical reactions: Advancing forward; directly penetrating; straight line movement.

Emotional reactions: Aroused; astonished; intensity; driven; focused; passionate; concentrating; dedicated; inspired.

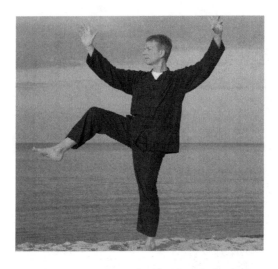

I would say that most people think of the Water, Air, or Earth movements as being most characteristic of Tai Chi. However, most popular Tai Chi sets include as many Fire reactions - and some sets even feature Fire reactions more than any other type.

Fire reactions often feature advancing movements and direct, straight line limb movement. You will often be stepping forward, while striking forward with the hand either as an open palm or as a fist.

It's easy to find examples in the Tai Chi sets of Fire movements that feature forward hand strikes. However, let's look at a rare example of Fire with a forward "foot" strike in the form of a kick.

In general, there are relatively few kicking movements in Tai Chi when compared to hand movements, and in fact some Tai Chi sets have no kicking at all. For the most part, the legs in Tai Chi are used as a stable base for hand and upper body movements. When the legs are used, they are used mostly to aid in felling your opponent in Air and Water reactions, or in stomping in Earth reactions.

For our example, let's look at the above movement, called *Right Separate Feet*. While some Tai Chi sets perform this kick with an Air (expanding) intention, the original movement is performed with an overwhelming Fire intention. The leg was lifted with the knee bent, and the kick is performed by swiftly unbending from the knee, with the toes kicking directly forward.

On a health level, Fire movements concentrate on more precise joint alignment - either in the arms (with a hand strike) or in the legs (with a kick). Whereas you can often "fudge" on the alignment in Water and Air arm movements, Fire movements require much more alignment and precision.

Fire movements relieve stress by developing one-pointed concentration and focus, allowing the brain and nervous system not to be distracted by the stressor and instead to keep your "eyes on the prize."

Air Reactions

Yin/yang: Greater yang.

Images: Hot air balloon; car air bag.

Physical reactions: Rising or lifting up; creating space or distance; expanding outward; forming a protective barrier.

Emotional reactions: Relaxed; calm; pensive; at ease; kind; gentle; unstressed; idealistic; expansive; open; free.

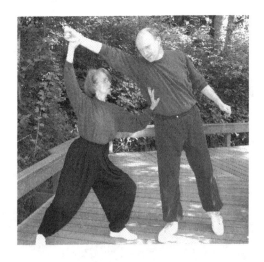

Air reactions are also quite frequent throughout most of the Tai Chi set. These movements generally feature opening and expansion throughout the body. They may include lifting or rising movements, or movements that create a large frame of "protective space" around the body.

Fan Through Back, shown on the left in the above photo, is a typical Air reaction. The player is just about to rise up and forward into her opponent, while at the same time maintaining protective space around her.

On the health level, Air movements help expand and open the body, increasing space in the internal body cavity. Given how as we age we tend to "collapse" into our torso, Air movement help to counteract that tendency. They also open our spine and joints, giving us greater flexibility and range of freedom in our movements.

Stress-wise, Air movements are about adding protective space around us. They are also about expanding our intention outward to the world around us, and giving us the compassion and insight to examine the world dispassionately, with kindness and calmness.

From Intention to Internal Power

As we mentioned several chapters ago, *"jin"* - in the physical Tai Chi sense - means using chi to generate power in movement to accomplish a certain goal. To this end, master have identified over 50 different *jin* in Tai Chi.

While many of these are extremely specialized, there are eight important *jin* that every Tai Chi student should at least be familiar with.

They are the so-called "Eight Jin" or "Eight Energies" of Tai Chi you may have heard about.

They are:

1. *Peng jin* ("Ward-off energy")

2. *Lu jin* ("Rollback energy")

3. *Ji jin* ("Press energy")

4. *An jin* ("Push energy")

5. *Cai jin* ("Pluck energy")

6. *Lie jin* ("Split energy")

7. *Zhou jin* ("Elbow energy")

8. *Kao jin* ("Shoulder energy")

The Four Primary Energies

In the last several chapters, we've explored four primary intentions in Tai Chi, which we called by the names of the Four Elements - Air, Water, Fire, and Earth.

But how do these Four Elements relate to these Eight Jin?

Quite simply, the Four Elements correspond to the first four of the Eight Jin.

The Ward-Off Energy of Air

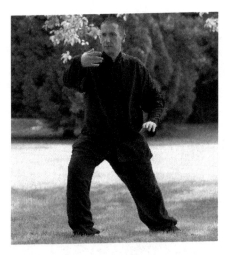

Our Air Element corresponds to *Peng jin* ("Ward-off energy"). The word "ward" means to protect, and the phrase "ward off" means to turn aside, to parry, and to prevent. In Tai Chi, this is mostly done through "expanding" intentions.

The primary purpose of Air Element patterns, whether we are practicing for health, stress relief, meditation, personal growth, or martial arts, is to expand our chi and have it flow through us and outward.

As an example of *Peng jin*, we can look at the Tai Chi movement named *Ward-Off*. (Note: "Ward-off" is both the name of a movement in Tai Chi as well as a *jin*. Keep in mind that many movements contain "ward-off *jin*", not just the one movement named "Ward-off".)

In the Tai Chi *Ward-Off* pattern, we are turning aside potential attacks and using our leading arm first to build a protective wall around us, and then to parry and redirect to the side.

The Rollback Energy of Water

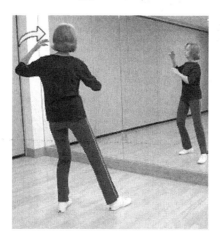

Our Water Element corresponds to *Lu jin* ("Rollback energy"). Rollback energy is used for retreating and protecting yourself, as well as gathering and collecting energy for your next outward expression. Often, you will be gathering the energy of an attack and easily dissipating it.

The primary purpose of Water Element response is to gather chi into us and redirect it to help us accomplish our goals.

As an example of *Lu jin,* we can look at the Tai Chi's *Rollback* pattern. (Once again, "Rollback" is both the name of a movement in Tai Chi as well as a j*in.* Keep in mind that many movements contain "rollback *jin*", not just the one movement named "Rollback".)

In this movement, you are taking an incoming attack and instead of resisting against it, you pull it towards you. By pulling the attack towards you rather than resisting, you will often gather the energy of the attack and easily dissipate it.

This may have the effect of unbalancing the attacker, as most attackers expect to be resisted, not aided, in their forward motion. So by pulling the attack towards you, you actually gain control of the attack. Once you have control, you can lead it harmlessly away and to the side of you.

The Press Energy of Fire

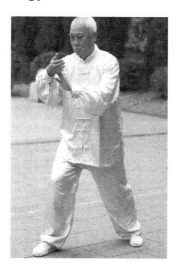

Our Fire Elements corresponds to *Ji jin* ("Press energy"). Press energy is used for direct attack forward in a martial situation. The primary purpose of Fire Element patterns is to express energy forward in a direct line.

As an example of *Ji jin*, we can look at the Tai Chi pattern that has the same name as the *jin, Press*. In the *Press* movement, you are expressing energy directly forward with either a strike or a trapping/squeezing movement.

Press is most often used against vulnerable areas in the body - that is, those areas not protected by bones or many layers of muscle. Striking to a vulnerable area protects us from injury to our hands, while at the same time allowing us to get the maximum effect with the minimum effort. Even a light strike or touch to a vulnerable area may have the effect of capturing your opponent's attention, stopping him and "unbalancing" him - psychologically and physically.

The Push Energy of Earth

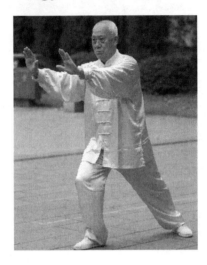

And finally, our Earth Element corresponds to *An jin* ("Push energy"). Unfortunately, in English the connotation of "push" is that you are pushing forward, as if you were pushing a door open, or pushing a stalled automobile. This connotation leads many students to think of Push as pushing forward (which is really *"Ji" jin*) or as expanding forward (which is really *"Peng" jin*).

Instead, in *An jin*, you are compressing energy downward into your attacker, attempting to uproot him. (Uprooting means to sever your opponents "roots" or connection to the ground.) Adding excess energy with a downward intention often "overburdens" the legs of your attacker, making him "weak-kneed."

If he does uproot upon the Earth movement, you can then add a Fire intention (to push him directly away) or an Air intention (to "launch" him away). However, this should only be done after the Earth energy has done the job of uprooting.

Again, as an example of *An jin,* we can look at the Tai Chi pattern that has the same name as the *jin, Push.* In the *Push* movement, you shift forward and push downward to overburden your attacker's support leg and uproot him.

Once you feels through your hands that he is uprooted, you may then follows with a slight Fire intention or Air intention to push the attacker away. By using a downward Earth compression to overburden an attacker's support leg, even a smaller, physically weaker person can "uproot" and push away a bigger, stronger person with a minimum of effort.

The Four Secondary Jin

So we've seen how our Four Elements actually correspond to the first four of the Eight Jin. But what about the remaining four?

These last four of the Eight Jin are seen as variations of the first four.

The Pluck Energy of Double Yin

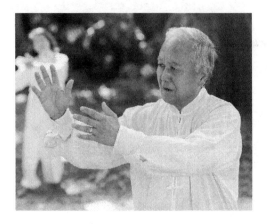

Cai jin ("Pluck energy") is a special combination of the yin Elements of Water/Rollback and Earth/Push Down, along with a specific "directional" intent when applying the Elements.

In a simple Water or Earth movement, you usually move your hands in the same/parallel direction. Think of the "Rollback" and "Push" Tai Chi movements we looked at above, where the arms are rolling back or pushing in the same general direction.

In *Cai jin* however, your arms move toward each other. The intent is to create a trapping or squeezing movement in which you are pushing together, as well as pulling in (Water) and/or pulling downward (Earth). The trapping is usually performed on an opponent's arm or other vulnerable body part.

If the movement mixes both Water/Rollback and Earth/Push Down in a direction toward each other, you'll create a "jerking" or "yanking" movement to pull the opponent down as well as towards you at the same time.

This combined Earth-and-Water *Cai jin* can be seen in the Tai Chi movement called "Play Pipa", pictured above. Your hands pull toward you with Water while also pulling down with Earth, with both hands squeezing toward each other.

The Split Energy of Double Yang

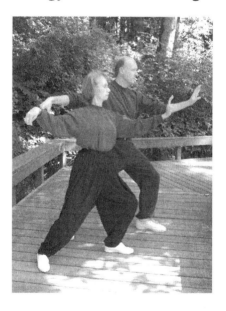

Lie jin ("Split energy") is a special combination of the yang Elements of Fire/Press and Air/Ward-Off, along with a special directional intent.

In *Lie jin*, you will be combining Fire and/or Air, but in two completely different - sometimes opposite - directions.

The key to *Lie jin* is that these two different directions have an equal intensity of yang. An Air movement like "Ward-Off" (described above under "Ward-off *Jin*") is **not** a split movement, even though the hands are moving in different directions. In "Ward-off", the lower hand is performing a yin Earth intention, and is acting as a counter-balance to the Air intention of the upper hand. Since the lower hand is in a supporting role, this type of movement is not truly a "Split" jin movement.

Instead, in a "Split" jin movement, the intention is two yang elements (Fire and/or Air) in two different directions, with equal intensity.

When Air is performed in two opposite directions, *Lie jin* creates an extreme opening of the body.

You can see this body opening in the Tai Chi movement called "Single Whip", pictured above. In Single Whip, both arms are performing Air movements in opposite directions. The creates one of the most open movement in any form of Tai Chi.

The Elbow and Shoulder Energies of Fire

Both of the last two energies, *Zhou jin* ("Elbow energy") and *Kao jin* ("Shoulder energy") are specialized forms of Fire/Ji Jin.

Whereas most Fire movements involves striking forward with the palm, fist, or foot, *Zhou jin* uses the elbow, while *Kao jin* uses the shoulder.

In addition to using different parts of the anatomy, what also makes these jin unique from standard Fire/Ji Jin movements is the situations in which they are used.

Usually, these jin occur during one of two situations:

1. Elbow/shoulder *jin* often occur after a Water, Earth, or *Cai jin* movement results in an opponent who is physically close to you. Because they are too close for a palm or fist strike, you may use your elbow or shoulder instead.

2. These elbow/shoulder *jin* may also be used after you've attempted a Fire palm or fist strike, but were unable to reach your opponent due to a block. Through re-positioning your arm and stepping closer to your opponent, you change from a palm strike to an elbow or shoulder strike.

In either situation given above, it's not unusual to start with either an elbow or shoulder strike, but switch to the other strike depending on what your opponent does. If you start with an elbow strike, but your opponent moves closer to you or attempts Earth jin on your elbow during your re-positioning, you may switch to a shoulder strike. Or if you start with a shoulder strike, but you opponent backs away with Water jin, you might switch to an elbow strike.

So from all of the above examples, you can see how easy it is to apply what you've learned in the Four Elements to understanding the Eight Jin. And as many masters have pointed out, these Eight Jin form the basis of understanding the expression of Chi in Tai Chi for both health and martial applications.

Structural Aspects of Internal Power

As we mentioned several chapters ago, physical definition of *jin* usually used in Tai Chi has two important parts: (1) using chi to generate power in movement, and (2) using the movement for a specific purpose.

In the last several chapters, we explored the second part of this definition, using movement for a specific purpose. We mentioned that there are over 50 different "intention-based" *jin* in Tai Chi, but we covered the eight most important *jin* identified by Tai Chi masters.

Now let's turn our attention to the first part of the definition of *jin* - using chi to generate power in movement.

The Skills You Need

As we mentioned, this first part of our physical definition of *jin* is the easiest to accomplish. Earlier in this book, in the earlier chapter entitled *Power: Internal Jin,* we give you a "kinesthetic experiment" that gives you the feeling of "chi-generated movement".

Of course, the movement we used in this experiment was extremely simple. It was only a movement of the arms, with none of the stepping, shifting, or turning found in most Tai Chi movements. In order to use chi to generated these more complex Tai Chi movements, you will need to develop several important skills.

These skills often spell the difference between your being able to generate *jin* or not. These skills also spell the difference between Tai Chi that gives you its full health, stress relief, and Chi Development benefits or not as well.

Jin in Combat vs. *Jin* for Health

Note that it is difficult to generalize about <u>all</u> the skills you might need for any of the 50+ *jin*. Some *jin* actually require opposite skills to perform. However, most Tai Chi masters specialize in only a handful of the *jin*. As you may have guessed, we have specialized in the four primary *jin* (the Four Elements) identified by masters in the Eight Jin list.

In my earlier days, when I was more martially oriented, I practiced these Four Elements *jin* specifically for martial applications. However, now that I'm older and nearing 60 years of age, my focus for these *jin* is now on health, stress relief, and Chi Development.

While the Four Elements *jin* have dual "health/martial" purposes, that is <u>not</u> true of all *jin*. Some *jin* - especially more martially oriented *jin* - may be extremely effective in combat, but are draining on your overall health and energy. However, the Four Element *jin* serve both purposes admirably.

So given the wide variety of *jin*, it's hard to identify all the skills you might need for any given *jin*. However, focusing on the Four Elements Jin, we can list the primary skills you'll need for more complex chi-generated movement. And these skills will serve you well in almost all jin, whether you are interested in martial jin or health jin.

Open Body Movement

Being able to move freely is required to issue internal power. Flexibility is somewhat important, but more importantly is range of motion in all the major joints of the body. Especially for Tai Chi, a loose and flexible waist, hips, and spine are required.

Deeper Layer Muscle Movement

To issue *jin*, you must be able to move in a relaxed fashion, and relying more on deeper layer muscles and less on the surface muscles most people use for movement.

Coordinated Movement

Two types of coordination are needed for *jin*. First, you'll need physical coordination that will teach you how to use your body in an integrated fashion. Secondly, you'll need to coordinate movement, breathing, and mental concentration to issue *jin*.

Structural Alignment

Keeping your muscles and bones in proper alignment during movement can be extremely difficult. But misalignment may cause chi to be locked and blocked in a part of the body, reducing *jin*.

Precision

The skill of "precision" is related to structural alignment, but at a more detailed level. For example, a few centimeters difference either way in limb or torso placement may not cause serious misalignment, but it may make the difference between success and failure in activating an energy pathway for *jin*.

Rooting

The technical definition of rooting is "a stable and stabilizing connection to the ground, both physical and energetic, such that any force you apply or any force applied to you does not unbalance you".

The term is a metaphor for the roots of a large tree, such as a mighty oak. Roots of these trees extend deep into the ground, providing the tree with stability. Rooting is important for issuing *jin* in Tai Chi.

Full Body Chi Connections

The goal here is to have an stable pathways of energy through your whole body. Ideally, these pathways is to help you create "unbroken threads" of energy that maintain the same intensity level through your body from start to finish in your movement.

A Strong Wei Chi

The chi in our body creates an energy field, called "Wei Chi" that actually extends out past your skin in all directions. The stronger this field, the more you will be able to issue *jin* outside your body.

Open Element Centers

Each of the Four Elements Jin rely on special energy centers within the body. Having these centers strong, stable, and "open" greatly improves your ability to create and issue *jin*.

Five Body Skills

In addition to these generalized skills, the Four Elements *jin* also requires special skills in five primary body parts.

1. The Legs

The legs are a major source of Four Elements *jin*. Generally, you will be using one leg like a coiled spring, then pushing downward with this leg to cause a rebound energy to bounce up the leg through the waist and into the hands.

2. Hips/Waist

In the Four Elements, the inner hip fold and waist play a major part in expressing *jin*. Hip and waist *jin* is usually started by the "rebound" jin of legs, but closing then opening the hips and waist adds an intensifying effect to the rebound.

3. Spine

Opening the spine also adds its own *jin* to any of the *jin* being issued by the legs and waist. And spinal alignment, including placement of the sacrum, is also crucial for the *jin* of the lower body to reach the shoulders and arms in Four Elements *jin*.

4. Shoulders

After the waist and spine, the shoulders are one place where chi often gets locked or blocked, hindering Four Elements *jin* expression. As such, I strongly recommend for both health and martial purposes, that you practice certain qigong exercises regularly to keep your shoulders open and loose.

5. Arms

Four Elements *jin* is mostly expressed through the elbows, wrists, and hands. That's why it is important to keep the chi pathways in the arms open.

Whether you practices for health, stress relief, martial arts, or Chi Development, the above structural skills are the primary ones you'll need for more complex chi-generated movement to reach your goals.

But how do you develop these skills?

The Chi Pyramid: Building Up to Jin

To help you develop *jin*, I'd like to share with you a particular "progression" we developed that has helped immensely with getting our students to generate, feel, and use chi.

This chi progression has been one of the biggest reasons for the benefits that many of you have gotten from our Tai Chi and Qigong programs. This progression has been our foundation. For example, our online ChiFusion™ program (which has over 4,500 members) is organized along the lines of this progression. It is in part why that program has been so long-lived, and so successful.

We came up with the first version of this chi development progression around 1999. It took us a number of years to refine it to its current form. But it is the one we've been using since 2004 or so, and it still stands to this day.

Results First

When we created this chi progression, our primary goal was results. We wanted our students to get results from their practice, and get them quickly.

Most of our students came to us to improve their health, recover from illness or injury, for gentle exercise, for stress relief, for mobility and flexibility, for balance, and to just plain get moving again. We didn't want them to wait months or years to see benefits to their health and well-being. We wanted something to happen within the first few weeks of practice.

Start Easily, But Build Quickly

But even though we wanted to show them some quick upfront results, we also wanted to start the students off easily.

We didn't want them to have to learn a lot of complicated movements or forms right at the beginning. We wanted simple chi movements – movements that were more like Western-style exercise or yoga, which they may already be familiar with. That would lower the "barrier to entry" for new students.

On the other hand, while we wanted them to start easily, we want them to build skills quickly. We wanted them to start becoming aware of chi, and have some skill in using it, within about four months - or sooner if possible.

After that initial foundation, we would introduce more advanced practices, such as energy threading, within 6 to 8 months. Finally, we would follow up with even more benefits-filled practices, like Four Elements-based chi practices, within 8 to 10 months.

In other words, our goal was to go from zero experience with Tai Chi or Qigong right to the heart of Chi Development in less than a year.

Efficient Skill Building

To do that, we had to focus on skills and benefits, and we had to be efficient. To make this work, we had to use as few movements as possible to teach the most important chi skills.

For example, if we could teach the same set of skills using five movements or ten movements, we would choose the five movements. Moreover, if we could teach one movement, but use it to build four or five different skills at the same time, that would be even better.

To do this though, we couldn't be "style-bound." We couldn't be loyal to a certain style, or a certain lineage, or a certain set of forms. We always had to be on the lookout for forms that fit in with the chi development progression and its goals. The chosen practices had to be both efficient (smaller number of movements to accomplish the goals) and effective (brought results).

We did a lot of experimenting to pick the Tai Chi and Qigong movements we finally chose. For example, those of you who've been in our online ChiFusion™ course know that in our first level, we teach Standing Eight Brocades. But what you may not know is that Eight Brocades was not our first choice for Level 1. It wasn't even our second choice. Or our third choice.

We tried three different styles to accomplish the Level 1 goals, before settling on the Eight Brocades. But these other styles all involved more than eight movements, whereas Eight Brocades (coupled with the unique details we brought to it) covered everything we wanted for that first level. So Eight Brocades won out, because of the fewer number of movements involved.

Speaking of details...

Many Details in Fewer Movements

We emphasized learning a small number of movements, mostly because we could be more efficient and help students get better results more quickly. But we also were guided by the idea that **it was better to do a few moves well, than hundreds of movements sloppily.**

To that end, we focused on *many details in fewer movements*, rather than fewer details in many movements. The more detailed we could make each movement, the more skills we could teach in each one. That way, our students could make the best use of their practice time.

The Five-Step Chi Pyramid

The chi development progression has five steps:

1. Open the Chi Meridian System and "Tune"the Body

2. Integrate Chi Meridians with Chi Vessels

3. Connect Managing Chi with Guardian Chi

4. Direct Chi through Four Intentions

5. Harmonize and Align Chi "Super Vessels"

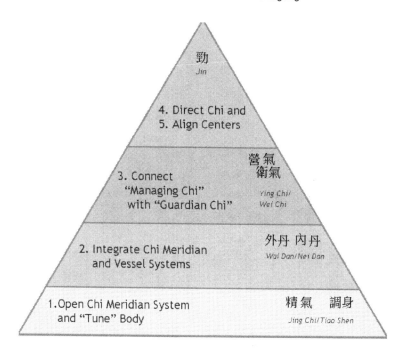

I've used this pyramid drawing to give you a good visual representation of how each step is built on the previous steps.

I've done this to show you that these aren't five random steps you can do in any order. There is definitely a progression that needs to be followed, since each step builds the foundation for the steps that follow.

1. Open the Chi Meridian System and "Tune" Body

This step focuses on the chi meridians. These are the pathways in the body that circulate chi.

To that end, we focus on two important skills in this level: (1) learning to circulate chi in the most efficient way possible, with a special focus on compensating for any problems with *chi dissipation,* and (2) learning to regulate the body according to the practices of *tiao shen* or "body tuning" that we discussed earlier in this book.

These two skills are intertwined. Good body tuning helps with chi circulation and prevents dissipating (wasting) chi that you generate during practice. So to that end, we focus most of our time on *tiao shen* - a set of skills that teach you how to use the body in an "energy efficient" manner.

For those of you who are in our online courses, you've seen and read about our "kinesthetic details" and our "ChiFusion™ details." These are all based on these physical and energetic *body tuning* practices.

To help with these skills, we focus on Waidan Qigong styles. The term *waidan* (pronounced "why don") means *external elixir.*

You can think of the word "elixir" as meaning chi. In this particular context, the word "external" means *external to the torso* - in other words, the arms and legs. Many important chi meridians are located in the limbs and have access points there. Waidan Qigong styles focus on these meridians, improving the flow of energy through them by focusing on moving the arms and legs.

One reason we chose Waidan Qigong styles for this level is that they are easier to learn. Waidan styles are more like

Western-style exercise, as compared to Neidan ("internal elixir" - pronounced "nay don") styles of qigong.

In addition, when you combine Waidan styles with body tuning, you often see faster progress up front, especially if you have health problems, illness, or injury.

Neidan styles, the other major division of Qigong alongside Waidan, are more of a "slow build" to health and chi. You'll see relatively little progress at first, but they provide many long term benefits. Waidan styles, on the other hand, are often more dramatic up front. While the Waidan benefits do tend to taper off after a time, a majority of students, including the sedentary and physically challenged, see short-term benefits more quickly this way.

As I mentioned earlier, we use Standing Eight Brocades for this level, but it's not the Brocades that really do the work. It's the body tuning details. Practically any Waidan style will work for this level, as long as you practice it with good body tuning.

2. Integrate Chi Meridians with Chi Vessels

This level focuses more on storing chi in the vessels. If you think of "vessels" like pots, urns, or vases, you get the idea of a container that holds something. That's what chi vessels are like. You can think of them as "holding tanks" or "reservoirs" for chi. Vessels are pathways where chi is stored, while meridians are pathways where chi is circulated.

So to focus more on chi vessels in this level, we use Neidan qigong styles. *Neidan*, as I mentioned above, means "internal elixir." "Internal" in this context refers to "inside the torso." Neidan Qigong styles focus on building up and storing energy in the torso, where most of the vessels are.

In addition to working on storage in this level, we also want to improve connections from the storage vessels to the chi-flow meridians. We do this by using Waidan/Neidan hybrid practices - that is, practices that combine elements from both styles.

By improving chi storage in your vessels, then improving how it is distributed to your meridians, you'll often create greater internal health, and see long term improvements and protection against chronic health problems.

The challenge here is that Neidan and Waidan/Neidan hybrid exercises are more complex to practice than Waidan exercises. So details become even more important at this stage.

3. Connect Managing Chi with Guardian Chi

In the first two steps, we focused on working with chi inside the body. This type of chi is called *Ying Chi* in Chinese - which means "managing chi" - because it manages all the functions inside the body.

But we also have chi outside of our body. Specifically we have a "chi field" that surrounds our body in all directions. This field is called *Wei Chi* (pronounced "way chi") in Chinese. That translates to "guardian chi," because it guards and protects us from pathogens and toxins in our environment. This includes not only physically harmful elements, but also mental and emotional "toxins" from stressful situations and people.

With our external guardian chi, we want to make sure that it can circulate freely and doesn't stagnate, just like the chi inside our body. We want to prevent blockages and discontinuities, so one of the main tasks in this step is to sense our external chi field, and find ways to keep it circulating. To do that, we learn to extend our internal chi outside of our body and connect it to this external chi.

To that end, we focus in this level on three skills: (1) *active rooting*, (2) whole body *energy threading*, and (3) bolstering the guardian Chi field.

Rooting is a common term in Tai Chi used to signify our ability to both physically and energetically connect to the ground or surface we are standing on.

The idea is that as you perform Tai Chi movements, you should remain balanced and stable - nothing you do should "uproot" you. However, most Tai Chi and Qigong students develop what we call "passive rooting" - that is, remaining stable by staying within certain limits and not overdoing. But here we focus on *active rooting* - by connecting your inner "managing" chi to the external "guardian" chi that extends into the ground.

Energy threading refers to developing unbroken, continuous threads of energy through the body. For example, we explore how to circulate guardian chi from below the feet and direct it up through your legs, then through your body, and out to your hands. This whole body threading can be used to detect blockages in your chi as a kind of "early warning system" to help you spot health problems before they become more serious.

Finally, we also work on detecting and strengthening the chi field that surrounds your body. We work on improving this chi field by actively circulating chi from our primary energy collector inside the body to the field outside the body, and back again.

Interestingly, we found that we could teach most of these skills, especially the energy threading and chi field strengthening, by using just one Tai Chi movement. No need for multiple movements or longer forms. These skills can be learned with just one Tai Chi movement.

For our courses, we chose a modified version of the *Cloud Hands* movement from Yang style Tai Chi, but there are another dozen Tai Chi movements from Yang and other styles that would have worked just as well.

4. Direct Chi through Four Intentions

By the time you've reached step four, you've now taken both your internal and external chi to higher levels. Once you've done that, it's time to learn to "do" something with the chi you've developed.

That's what the final two levels are about. In the pyramid drawing, I've put steps four and five together, since they are related. But let's discuss step four first.

This fourth level is where we reach the level of working on *jin*. This is the level where we focus on the Four Elements and four primary intentions in Tai Chi. Plus you are learning how to develop whole-body chi health by expressing these Chi Elements through movement.

5. Harmonize and Align Chi "Super Vessels"

Over the centuries, various disciplines both East and West have identified special energy centers in the body.

The number of these energy centers vary from anywhere from three to twelve or more. For example, the Hindu yoga system identifies seven chakra (their name for these centers), while Buddhist systems and some Western systems identify five energy centers.

Keep in mind, there is no "correct" or "true" system here. These are all just models, and you can use three, four, five, six, ten, twelve, or a hundred energy centers - whatever is most useful to what you are trying to accomplish.

For our work, we chose to focus on five energy centers. These five special chi centers are like *super vessels* as far as chi storage is concerned. But unlike the regular chi vessels that are just inside the body, these five centers include three inside the body and two outside the body.

Through movement, mental concentration, breathing, and focus, you charge, align, and connect these centers to unleash vast amounts of healing energy.

These centers are directly tied to the four Tai Chi elements/intentions of *air, fire, water,* and *earth,* along with a special center for the *spirit/void.*

Working through this pyramid helps you develop the necessary physical prerequisites for developing *jin,* as well as helps instill both the mental and energetic intention you'll need for strong chi development.

Congratulations

Congratulations on completing this book on *The Four Treasures of Tai Chi and Qigong.*

I hope that you now have a better understanding of *jing, chi, shen* and *jin* in Tai Chi and Qigong

We've covered a lot of the theory behind Tai Chi and Qigong. I realize this theoretical material is sometimes difficult to understand. However, if you reinforce this material through practice, I think you'll find more benefits by "experiencing" these concepts rather than just reading about them.

If you would like to really boost your experience with more advanced approaches to Qi Development, you would benefit greatly from our *Qi Masters* program.

To help you explore more deeply into the physical, mental, emotional and energetic aspects of Tai Chi and Qigong, please visit us online at **www.QiMasters.com.**

And thank you again for purchasing this book and supporting our work. We appreciate having dedicated students like you who show their support.

As always, you have my best wishes for success in Tai Chi, Qigong, and Chi Development.

Al J. Simon

Complimentary Bonuses Just For You (a $97 Value)

I have some special bonuses exclusively for you as a reader of *The Four Treasures of Tai Chi and Qigong.*

Just go online to www.QiTreasures.com/bonuses and you can download the following:

✓ **Wenji Qiwu Qigong - An Exercise for Mind, Body, and Chi Integration (five online videos, photos, and written instructions)**

Wenji Qiwu (pronounced like "when-jee chee-woo") Qigong is a simple, one-movement Qigong practice.

The name literally means "hear rooster, raise, wield". But more figuratively, it means "Rise in the morning to perform the sword dance" though there is no sword involved. It is an easy movement that doesn't take much time to learn. In addition, it's done standing in place, so it doesn't require much space for practice.

This calming movement works on the energy pathways associated with mind and body integration. But it is also great for overall physical health, as well as mental and emotional stress relief.

This simple, single movement practice is not only easy to learn, it's easy to master. So you can more quickly go from having to concentrate on the movements, to allowing the movements to happen, the mind to relax, the body to open, and the chi to flow.

But don't let its simplicity fool you. This power of this qigong movement will help you get more chi from your existing Tai Chi or Qigong practice. It will allow you to better integrate your movements with the flow of chi you will feel.

You'll get over 19 minutes of video plus written instructions and photos to cover all the details of this one qigong movement.

✓ **Huangying Diebang (Oriole Flaps Wings) Qigong (five online videos, photos, and written instructions)**

Huangying Diebang (pronounced like "wong-ying dee-yea-bong") in Chinese means something like "bright yellow bird folds arms," but it's usually translated as "oriole flaps its wings."

This particular standing-in-place movement opens the chi energy points and pathways that are associated with a calm, receptive state of mind.

This calm state of mind is a particular important requirement for deeper chi development. But don't think of calm as the opposite of "active." Think of calmness as a middle ground between agitated and active on one side, and passive and inactive on the other. Calm is being mentally aware and alert, but not emotionally aroused. It's being emotionally even, but still focused on a mental level.

In addition to calm mental states, this qigong drains stagnant chi from the upper limbs with its unique "flapping" motions. It stimulates the internal organs by using the back of the arms to press or massage over the kidneys in the back. In addition, the stance opens the legs and the acupuncture points in the perenium to facilitate chi flow to the legs.

All of these features of this exercise contribute to developing the mental and emotional states that facilitate deeper chi development.

You'll get 23 minutes of video plus written instructions and photos to cover all the details of this one qigong movement.

✓ **"Guided Ripple" Tai Chi (three online audios, video, photos, and written instructions)**

This set of three audios helps you sense and connect into the chi energy field that surrounds you. You'll experience how your body and intention can cause ripples in this energy field, and how you can use these ripples to create movement.

For this practice, we use a very simple Tai Chi movement called "Lifting Water" or "Raise Hands." If you already know this movement from Tai Chi, that's great, but in case you don't, I've included instructions for the movement.

Once you have this simple movement down, you'll learn how to perform it using ripples in the energy field that surrounds you. You'll learn how to create ripples simply through your intention, then allow those ripples to create the movements. Eventually, you'll learn to sense ripples that are already in the field - from other objects, people, events, situations, thoughts, even emotions - and allow those ripples to create the movement.

It's a fascinating experience of allowing the chi energy field to move you rather than you merely moving through the field.

You'll receive a short video and written instructions on how to perform Tai Chi's "Lifting Water" movement. Then you can use the three audios (each one is eight to twelve minutes in length) to experience the movement, intention, and sensation of using chi energy field ripples to create the movement.

You can download these special bonuses online from this web page: www.QiTreasures.com/bonuses

I hope you'll accept these bonuses as my thank you for reading this book. It's one of the ways I go the extra mile to show my appreciation for your support.

As always, I wish you the best for your health, well-being, and happiness.

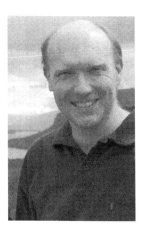

About the Author

Al Simon is a certified Tai Chi and Qigong master. He is the "founding father" of online Tai Chi and Qigong instruction. He was the first master to teach online in 2003, and he now has 4,500 online students all over the world.

Al Simon learned his first Qigong exercises in 1975. He studied Zen meditation in 1982 and began Tai Chi in 1984.

He received certification from Master Lawrence Galante, author of the book *Tai Chi - The Supreme Ultimate*. Al is also mentioned in the book *Mastering Yang Style Tai Chi*.

Al has been inducted into the United States Martial Arts Hall of Fame three times. Al was inducted with the **rank of "Master"** by the International Martial Arts Headfounders Grandmasters Council. He was also inducted with the **rank of "Founder"** for the development of the ChiFusion™ program.

Al is also the author of the books, *50 True Chi Stories; To Float Like Clouds, To Flow Like Water; Three Monk Mindfulness;* and *Start From Zero.*

Al appeared as a guest on both season one and season two of the *Living Energy Secrets* series, as well as BlogTalk Radio's *Secrets of Qigong Masters.* In addition, Al's articles on Tai Chi, Qigong, and Chi Development have appeared in publications such as *Wholistic Alternatives, Natural Health Newsletter, The Empty Vessel,* and *Chi Journal.* His Chi Development program was also spotlighted on Shirley MacLaine's *Independent Expression Radio* show.

Al is also a member of Mensa, the high I.Q. society.

Your Invitation

Want to learn more advanced approaches and practices in Chi Development?

We invite you to join us as we explore how to break through to higher levels of health, stress relief, vitality, energy, and power in your Tai Chi and Qigong practice.

For support in taking your next steps towards higher levels in your Tai Chi and Qigong, please visit us online at:

www.QiMasters.com

Made in the USA
San Bernardino, CA
29 October 2018